Your Guide To Gay Bathhouses

Bathhouse Blues

I have tried to recreate events, locales, and conversations from my memories. To maintain people's anonymity, I have changed the names of individuals and places in some instances. I may have changed some identifying characteristics and details, such as physical properties, occupations, and places of residence.

ISBN: 979-8-224-78485-1

PRAISE FOR BATHHOUSE BLUES

"This anonymous web author's essays are worth a browse. Be advised that it's all straight-talking expository dialogue, earnest and in some cases, a bit wide-eyed. Still, the author's intentions are noble."
➢ Unzipped Magazine

"What a good effort here to educate and enlighten people on an area that is little known by outsiders - the gay bathhouse. Recommended."
➢ Jane's Guide

"Bathhouse Blues is the best thing I've read about the sexual politics of gay sex in a semi-public arena."
➢ Tablet Magazine

"These stories may not get you off, but they provide a fascinating characterization of a system that many gay men draw themselves into without really knowing why."
➢ Dark Post

"A well written and entertaining site packed with exciting stories and information, whether you are a bathhouse regular, or have always wondered what goes on in these places. The author delves into pretty much every topic you can imagine associated with 'The Tubs.'"
➢ Search The Gay Web

MORE TITLES BY THIS AUTHOR

No Asians Please
How Asian Men Get Perceived In The Gay
Community

Gay Steam
True Sex Tales From The Tubs

Back To The Baths
More Gay Bathhouse Stories

DEDICATION.

To Bjorn, Michael, and Lloyd.

The European, Canadian, and American.

Without you, I wouldn't have made it this far.

Thank You.

INTRODUCTION

I am a gay Asian male who has written a gay bathhouse blog called Bathhouse Blues. These are my experiences and observations in a gay bathhouse setting for over 20 years. This book represents the best and most educational stories about bathhouse culture.

Let me provide some background information. I've been visiting the baths for over twenty years, starting when I was 21. Typically, I visit the baths once a week. Occasionally, I go two or three times a week. I have gone at all hours—morning, noon, evening, or late at night. Through those visits, I have met some of the most diverse and exciting people. I've had wonderful conversations with men I've never met before, observing phenomena I didn't know existed, like bukkake, Glory Holes, and even open drug use. Now I want to share what I have witnessed.

I started writing these stories because I realized no one has ever written about what happens inside a bathhouse. You can find many erotic stories written about sensual encounters in the baths. However, the sexual politics and culture within a bathhouse remain unexplored. It is a whole other world. I hope that by writing about these topics, people can gain a deeper understanding of the gay community. We shouldn't regard it as a taboo term.

I will not tell you who I am or where I live. I will say that these essays originate in a vast urban North American city with an extensive and diverse gay community. I encourage the reader to use their imagination when reading these stories, as the setting could be any city, regardless of size, and the bathhouse experiences are universal.

I hope to entertain, educate, and open your eyes to new perspectives.

These are my stories.

Me.

TABLE OF CONTENTS

CHAPTER 1
Gay Bathhouse Etiquette

First and foremost, bathhouses are places for men to have sex. It serves as a sexual playground where men can indulge in their desires and engage in sexual activities around the clock, akin to a 24-hour convenience store. Come to think of it, the baths are like a supermarket. You can shop for whatever you are looking for. In a bathhouse, you can choose from Latinos to Twinks, Bears to Chubs, Asians to Blacks—whatever type of guy you are interested in, you will find. Far more than bars or clubs, the baths have something for everyone.

There are two misconceptions about bathhouses. First, only dirty older men go to the baths. Second, only gorgeous men can get lucky at a bathhouse. Neither is true. As I mentioned at the start, there is something for everyone. Sometimes, men use the baths to find a specific "type" of guy they can't find anywhere else, such as an Asian, Chub, Bear, and so on.

Bathhouses can be found in various locations, ranging from a side street to an obscure neighborhood. Most times, there is no sign on the door. You walk in and see a cashier located behind a protective window. The wall will display the list of prices for purchasing a room or a locker. Renting a room will give you privacy. If you choose to rent a locker, which is less expensive than a room, you won't have any privacy, especially if you happen to meet someone attractive. Most bathhouses will allow you to lock up your valuables in a safe—like a watch, wallet, or jewelry. Once you pay, the cashier will buzz you in, and you can open the door. The door will automatically close behind you. There is no chance of any strangers walking in by accident.

Depending on where you live, you might be required to purchase a bathhouse membership. The reason? According to some state laws, a bathhouse can only operate as a private men's club. Therefore, each patron must possess a membership. Some bathhouses may only need you to fill out some information on a card. Other bathhouses, however, may request a photo ID. Whether you are in the closet or openly out, you needn't worry about your personal information being leaked.

To be profitable, bathhouses need customers. How would they be able to keep customers if they leak personal information? Not to worry, as bathhouses are very discreet when it comes to maintaining membership confidentiality. Therefore, you need not fear exposure. The upside is that memberships may also offer discounts if the customer plans on making multiple visits to the baths. After years of going to my regular bathhouse, I have recently purchased a membership. Since I go so often, it allows me to save money. Every bathhouse does not require a membership purchase. However, if your local bathhouse requires you to buy one, be prepared.

After arriving, undress, wrap the towel around your waist, and cruise. It would be best if you showered before you explored the hallways. That way, you are fresh for whoever you next encounter. Then, after you have done the deed, take another shower. This way, you can refresh yourself for the next guy you find. For some, taking three to five showers is not uncommon! That's how many times some guys get lucky at the baths. Some men are paranoid about foot fungus and bring slippers or sandals to protect their feet.

The baths consist of dozens of rooms, all lined up among a maze of hallways. You spend most of your time walking the halls looking for a score. Everyone knows why the other person is there. Guys lie in their rooms, observing other men as they pass by. Or they stand in the hallways, observing those who walk around them. Everybody is cruising everyone. There is even a bulletin board for people to advertise themselves. For example, the board displays the message, "Room 218, submissive bottom, shoot your load inside me." There are dozens of similar messages on the board.

All bathhouses will have a sauna, steam room, and multiple showers to clean up. Many will have a hot tub or a swimming pool, with some places having both. To pass the time, most have porno rooms. Condoms are free of charge, but you will have to pay for lube. Every bathhouse has a snack bar and a payphone. There is also a lounge area where you can sit and watch television. You can also enjoy reading gay magazines like Advocate and Instinct.

The rules are straightforward at the baths. You will know right away if someone likes you. They will make eye contact with you. If he initiates eye contact and you reciprocate, you can predict the outcome. Some guys will not make eye contact or even look away. You cannot take it personally. That is the most important bathhouse rule, but many find it challenging to understand.

What if an individual initiate's eye contact with you, and you are interested? Try stroking your dick or playing with your nipples. Touching can also be a helpful cruising tool. If you are sitting near someone, you may want to try playing footsies or reaching over and pinching his nipple. If you pass someone in the hallway, you may decide to have your hand brushed against him. Some older men will even be bold enough to grab a guy's crotch! You can do this light touching to gauge someone's interest. But don't throw yourself at him. That makes you look desperate, which is a turn-off for most men. If the guy turns and pushes you aside, walk away. Do not prolong the agony of trying to create something that will not happen. He is not interested.

If someone approaches you, that is not up to your standards; be gentle in turning him down. Remember the treatment you would expect. We have all been the recipients of rejection at one time or another. I usually tell guys that I am just walking around to get a feel for the place. If you want to be direct, say, "I am not interested." Do not say, "Get out of my face." That is rude, although you will come across guys who are that blunt.

Conversely, if someone turns you down, move on gracefully. Do not stalk the person and hang around outside his room. It makes him uncomfortable and makes you look like a fool. By obsessing over someone who is not interested, you might miss out on someone who is interested in you. That's why you move on when someone says, "No thanks."

When you begin exploring the rooms, you will find men lying on their beds in various positions. Lying face down means he wants anal. Sitting up could indicate a variety of intentions, but most likely it's just enjoyment. Kneeling on the floor, he says he wants oral. If you pass by a room and the guy looks away, it indicates a lack of interest. However, if he looks at you and starts stroking himself, you know where that will lead.

If you see two guys getting it on, wait for a signal that you can join in. A wink, nod, or even a hand wave is a signal. If there are no indications, they are not interested in a third party. They will gently or forcefully push you away if you try to join in. That is embarrassing, so wait for the signs.

Remember, this is a bathhouse where rejection happens every second. Therefore, you cannot take it personally; that is how it is. If you cannot accept that, the baths are not for you. If you leave with anything after reading these essays, leave with this. A bathhouse is a place where quickie sex is the norm. If you are looking for a long bonding experience with someone, you will not find that at a bathhouse. I am not saying that it cannot happen, but it is rare. Most times, at the baths, a man's focus is to get off and move on. It is the norm in a bathhouse environment for a guy to get up and leave—all within 30 seconds of reaching ejaculation.

Often, there is no exchange of pleasantries before or after sex. It wastes time because both of you are there—**FOR THE SEX!** So why spend time talking? Time and time again, a guy will get up, put his towel back on, and leave your room once the sex finishes, all without saying a word. Afterward, you may run into him roaming the hallways, looking for his next encounter. Some guys are insensitive enough to act like they've never seen you before. Again, you cannot take it personally. Gay bathhouses aim to facilitate effortless and speedy sexual encounters. You are not there to make friends. Some guys don't even stick around looking for round two. Satisfied by getting off, some immediately leave the baths. It is not rare for men to spend only 20 minutes on the premises. Why stay if they've achieved their goal of getting laid? But some guys in the closet feel guilty after having quickie sex. They find it cheap and sordid. These men run out of the baths guilt-ridden, vowing never to return. But that only lasts a few hours, and they return to the baths the next day.

I frequently receive the question, "Can you go to the baths as only an observer? Can you observe without attracting attention?" The answer is yes, and here is how you do it. Avoid undressing. No rule says you have to strip off all of your clothes. Being fully dressed is a sign to other men that you are off-limits. When customers see someone fully dressed, they assume that the person works at the baths. All patrons know the bathhouse staff is off-limits. My friend Ari will do just that. When he goes to the baths, he stays fully clothed, sits in a well-lit part of the bathhouse, and watches people pass by. No one bothers him. If Ari sees someone attractive, he will pursue his object of desire while fully clothed.

Above all, ensure your safety by using condoms and lube. Someone told me something that has stayed with me, which I will pass on to you. Do not do anything that you do not want to do. It is not worth it. Often, you will experience intense feelings of passion. Avoid feeling compelled to participate in risky sexual activities or anything that causes you discomfort, even for a brief moment. Around the corner, another guy will do what you want to do. So be patient.

I would like to offer my final advice on the Gay Baths.

Have Fun!

CHAPTER 2
Why Gay Men Go To The Baths

All these bathhouse stories probably have you asking, "Why do I spend so much time at the gay baths?" That is a fair question. This essay will clarify why so many gay men (me included) spend so much time at a gay bathhouse.

The bathhouse scene is a real society with its own rules, culture, and politics. No one has written about this unique world—until now. There is one thing the gay baths provide that no other gay establishment can offer: total acceptance. Let's face it: the gay community is very segregated and superficial. If you are a gym bunny, you belong in the circuit scene. If you're a Twink, you belong in the nightclub and bar scene. If you identify as a bear, it's the leather scene, and vice versa. You'd have a difficult time finding a gay senior or a visible minority in any of these environments.

The baths are the only queer meeting place where you can see a cross-section of every gay group imaginable—all under the same roof. On any night, you can see Latinos and Twinks, Bears and Chubs, Asians and Blacks, even Gay Seniors: all nationalities, all ages, and all shapes and sizes. There is acceptance for everyone, and no one faces rejection at the door.

Being practically naked makes you vulnerable and inhibited. When individuals remove their clothing, their barriers and defenses crumble. It establishes an equal and fair environment for men to engage with each other. No one knows the other person's profession or status, as everyone is in a towel. You may witness interactions between corporate lawyers and truck drivers, among others. The inequality aspect of the baths happens when everyone is naked, as some men are better looking than others.

Although the gay baths do not turn away anyone at the door, men still face judgment based on their appearance. But you have a better chance of meeting someone at the baths than at a bar or club. That is because bathhouses cater to different types of men. In contrast, bars and clubs cater to a specific type of man—twinks, bears, muscle men, etc. Men with similar characteristics would pack the venue. In short, bathhouses offer more variety, giving you better chances to meet someone.

Both baths and bars are superficial, but gay baths are more honest because everyone is naked. There is nothing to hide. In a bar, everyone highlights their appearance, and clothing can conceal an individual's imperfections. Despite mainstream advances, gay people can still feel isolated in the gay community. The baths allow men to mix with other gay men from all walks of life. It fills a need to connect with someone—one more reason why so many gay men go to the baths. What drives this desire? One word: loneliness, or rather, a subconscious feeling of isolation.

In reality, the desire to connect with another gay man drives the need for sex in the gay community. The sexual act fills the loneliness and the need for companionship, whether a quick blowjob or anal intercourse. That is why a lot of sex occurs in a bathhouse. What's the bottom line? There are a lot of lonely gay men in the world.

But many gay men go to the baths looking for some companionship in a non-sexual way. That is why you see more straight, married, bi, or closeted men at the baths. These men don't have many interactions with the gay community. But they need to connect in some way with other gay men. Whether they're engaging in a conversation or witnessing two gay men enjoying a quickie, it satisfies their desire to interact with other men. These men feel safer connecting with other gay men at the baths than in bars or clubs, as it is a closed-door environment. Bathhouses offer these men a false sense of security and acceptance. They experience a sense of liberation, allowing them to express themselves without restraint.

But it's not just these straight men who need to connect. Many gay men are lonely and need to communicate with other gay men. That is why you see the same men repeatedly at the baths. Think of a regular customer at a bar, and you get the idea—that sheer subconscious feeling of loneliness and a need to make a connection no matter how superficial.

Fortunately, my bathhouse is known for its friendliness, which has inspired these stories. All of the regular customers are warm and welcoming. In short, it is not only a sexual atmosphere but a social one. That social aspect is why men go to this particular bathhouse. Free sex is a secondary reason. Typically, this bathhouse stands out due to its unique approach. Also, you do not have to restrict yourself to doing just one thing. In the absence of conversation, you can do other things. You can sit in the sauna and steam room, relax in the whirlpool, read magazines in the lounge, watch TV or porn flicks, and chat with other guys. There is something for everyone.

When you start seeing the same men over and over again, conversations do begin to take place. Friendships can develop. However, it's important to keep in mind that these relationships are superficial. Once you leave the gay baths, you never see these men again until your next bathhouse visit. If you run into them again at the baths, you quickly pick up the conversation where you last left off. That could have been a week ago or six months ago. For instance, I was chatting in the lounge with another friend. Numerous men were passing by, and I had the opportunity to say hello to several of them. I knew all of them—15 in all. But I'm experienced enough to know that these relationships are not real. They don't go outside of the bathhouse environment.

If you know relationships at the baths are superficial, that's great. Unfortunately, many men mistakenly believe that a relationship develops at the baths. This misconception can lead to serious consequences. Plus, not all bathhouses are friendly, as conversation is practically nonexistent at other bathhouses. The majority of them are rather cold and uninviting. For instance, a different bathhouse in my city draws the most stunning men, each appearing as if they've stepped straight out of Men's Health magazine. But glance at any of these men, and they'll verbally rip you apart. The atmosphere is intense, with the guys solely focused on getting laid, viewing sex as a clinical and robotic activity. Many bathhouses are similar.

Therefore, because of its friendliness, I keep going to this particular bathhouse (not the one with the gorgeous men). I have been a loyal customer for decades, and I go for the escape. After a long day, it is lovely to get away from everything. Have a steam or sauna, dip in the whirlpool, and chat with someone. No one in your life will bother you. Cell phones, emails, and texts are nonexistent. You are free from the world. I'll be in the bathhouse lounge, totally naked in a towel, watching the news. Coffee and a roaring fireplace are beside me. I look out of the window and see it is raining. I am immersed in an escape world, hidden behind closed doors, while the real world is depicted on TV.

The irony does not escape me.

CHAPTER 3
Racism Or Preference At The Baths

The first two entries were to lay down a foundation for these stories. Right now, I'd like to tell you a bit about myself. Even though I am in my thirties, I still look a decade younger. People always ask me, "What are you taking in college?" or "Do you go to school?" when they meet me for the first time. I have this youthful, boyish face. Just last week, someone thought I was 23. It has gotten to the point that whenever someone asks me about my age, I usually reply, "Guess."

I have a short haircut and dimples on both cheeks. I just have an okay body, nobody's perfect. One person described me as having a down-home, apple-pie stoic sweetness about myself. However, when I'm at the baths, the other guys tend to ignore me 99.9% of the time—not giving me any attention. Given my description, one might assume that I would attract a large number of men. So why would I have this problem? Because I'm Asian. Gay men of any color, including Asians, are completely invisible to all men of white ethnicity.

There is still a racism problem in this country, which is most apparent in the gay community. Today's racism isn't blatant; instead, it is subtle. People often overlook this subtle form of discrimination. But every minute of every day, discrimination against people of all nationalities occurs. We all do it, and no one is immune. The most ironic thing about the gay community is that we have fought for equality in mainstream society. Yet, in many different settings, I've observed many gay men discriminate against each other.

The baths are like a microcosm of a small town that consists of only gay men. It's where you can see every gay group imaginable—all under the same roof. No other gay environment can offer such a wide variety of gay men interacting and playing sexual politics with one another. You will always see different types of men hooking up with each other on any given night, such as Chubs and Twinks, Bears and Smoothies, Gym Bunnies and Trans, etc. Despite these apparent differences, they all have one thing in common. All of these couples would be white. At the baths, you will see a wider variety of men together than an interracial pair.

Gay white men don't call this racism. Instead, they call it a preference. They say physical and sexual attraction is not racial or racist. Being unable to work with, be friends with, or do anything with a visible minority is racist. Does the fact that gay men don't find women attractive equate to sexism? Of course not. That is how gay white men rationalize their preference.

All gay men harbor a deep yearning for white men, a desire that stems from the constant barrage of male images in the media. They all contribute the same subliminal message, from grocery store checkout magazines to billboards along the highways: **WHITE IS BEAUTIFUL**. Gay white men have conditioned themselves to exclusively attract and associate with only their race. It has become a subconscious preference. Take this analogy. All gay men embrace their sexual orientation and only find attraction in other men. It is not a choice, as we were all born that way. Gay white men naturally gravitate toward their own race, just as gay men cannot control their attraction to other men. Thus, it is a preference.

Many gay white men will only talk to and associate with each other at the baths, even on a social level. For example, I have written about a Russian man who I often encounter at the baths. Due to his closeted status, he is eager to establish non-sexual connections with other gay men. I have witnessed him engaging in conversation with every white man at the baths, regardless of their age, weight, or complexion—the list is endless. He has talked to everyone except me and other visible minorities at the baths. I have **NEVER** seen him talk with anyone of a different color. We have never exchanged one word, yet we've seen each other at the baths weekly for years. We have even been in the whirlpool together, and he never speaks to me. However, whenever a white guy, or even a newcomer, joins the pool, the Russian guy initiates a conversation with them right away. There have also been a few times when he has ignored me right to my face. When I'm conversing with a white acquaintance, he approaches and initiates a conversation with that individual without acknowledging my presence or even saying hello. Then he will leave, bidding farewell to my white acquaintance, and I will remain completely invisible to him. Let me assure you, he is not the only one. Many other white guys at the baths have also treated me like I'm non-existent, despite standing in front of their faces. So, shyness is not an excuse.

The problem lies in the subtle racism. The Russian probably doesn't even think what he is doing is wrong. He's not advocating for people of color to sit in the back of the bus, making him racist. Many gay white men have never interacted with or grown up with people of color. Therefore, many people subconsciously hold the belief that all visible minorities are invisible. Gay white men only see other gay white men, period.

99.9% of the gay population (Gay White Men) find me undesirable, invisible, and worthless. So, where does that leave me as a visible minority? Not much.

These days, when I go to the baths, I observe and am a voyeur. You might wonder, "Why don't I hook up with a gay Asian male?" Visible minorities have the same ability to exhibit racism toward their own races. Their actions reflect those of their white counterparts toward a different racial group.

I cannot speak for other visible minorities, but I can talk about how gay Asian men can be racist against their own race. Similar to gay white men's subliminal preferences, most gay Asian men express an exclusive attraction toward white men. Asians' oppressive upbringing, which only involves attending school and studying at night, accounts for this. In adulthood, many Asians have major self-esteem issues. They lack the necessary social skills and maturity. In short, many gay Asian men continuously seek approval. I refer to this as the constant pursuit of approval, also known as the "disease to please." Many don't even identify as a different race, shielded from blatant racism growing up. Gay Asian men are oblivious to bigotry, thinking the world is one big, joyful family.

Since gay Asian men identify with white culture, it is natural they only want white sex. It is pathetic to watch gay Asian men chase after gay white men at the baths. Underneath this desire for white sex is an inherent, repressed inferiority. Gay Asian men attempt to fill their low self-esteem by hooking up with gay white men, as if white sex is superior. These gay Asian men, who want to please a gay white man, can receive the approval and acceptance they desperately crave. Despite that moment's fleeting nature, the path to achieving that security is temporary. Hooking up with a fellow Asian cannot fill the same emptiness of insecurity. Many Asians feel disgusted when interacting with or even glancing at other Asians. Gay Asian men who feel this way need to look in the mirror. Those feelings of disgust are actually feelings of insecurity and low self-esteem.

The worst part is that white men are fully aware of the attraction Asians have for them. This is likely the reason they treat Asians as "backups" at the baths. They can hunt for different prey, and if that hunt fails to find anyone, they come looking for the Asian guy waiting in the wings, ready to give a head. Unfortunately, this is the stereotype that many people hold about gay Asians. We are desperate, submissive, and subservient, willing to do whatever it takes to please. We Asians perpetuate that stereotype because we appear desperate for white love. But it can backfire. Some gay white men have said they would have considered hooking up with a gay Asian male. But the desperation is such a turn-off. This explains why some gay white men avoid any gay Asian men they might come across at the baths.

Given that 99.9% of the gay population rejects entire racial groups, what should a gay Asian man do? Embrace the next best option—an older white man. Gay Asian men are so obsessed with white men that even a 65-year-old is considered a catch. They see it as a status symbol, boosting their cachet within gay Asian circles. For some, it is a social-climbing function whereby a gay Asian man hopes to improve himself, like some gold-digging female. I am amazed by the sheer number of older white men who accompany very young Asian men, whether strolling down the street or at the baths. It is astounding. Older gay white men enjoy the attention from Asians. Indeed, it doesn't matter to older white men if the guy is green, as long as he's young and attractive. Given the prevalence of the "disease to please" among gay Asian men, many older gay white men take advantage of this situation.

Being with a young gay Asian male allows these older men to recapture a bit of their youth. We (Gay Asian Men) have a youthful appearance regardless of age. Another quality is our soft, smooth skin, which is a delight to touch. Additionally, Asians are, by reputation, very passive, subservient, and submissive in bed (in short, desperate). So, everyone's happy. Even though he's 65 years old, being white is the most important thing for a gay Asian man. At the same time, it is the perfect relationship! I genuinely believe that if any of these older men took a pill to turn 21, their interest in Asians would wane.

I calculated the number of men who expressed a genuine liking for Asians in their comments on my website. 97% were all over the age of 58— some even over 70! I have never had any white guy in their twenties or thirties (who did not admit to being a rice queen) disagree with me about their turn-off of Asians. **NOT ONE!**

It hurts me to see gay Asian men aligning themselves with older gay white men in this way. The stereotype that portrays us as gold-digging men who are only interested in gay white men, regardless of their age, unfairly lumps all other gay Asians together. Older gay white men hit on me almost every week at the baths. This is primarily due to my Asian ethnicity.

You, as a gay Asian male, may be reading this essay and saying it isn't true. However, think about it. How come no white guy in the gay community ever notices you at a bar, supermarket, or bookstore? Why do the white patrons immediately get up and leave when Asians enter the pool, sauna, or porn lounge at the baths? When you approach any white male participating in group sex activities, they tend to push you away. Depending on the situation, they may push you away gently or forcefully. Did you ever wonder why all the white gym guys are friendly to each other? But never talk to us Asians? Despite the fact that everyone's gaydar is operating at full capacity, why are we being ignored? Gay Asians are invisible and undesirable to the gay white community, not intentionally but subconsciously.

The rejection from numerous gay men can lead to anger and bitterness. You could also say, "We do not accept that!" We do not have to allow superficial gay white men to exploit us. We, as gay Asian men, must eliminate the stereotype of desperately chasing after gay white guys. We need to have more self-respect. Think of it as an iron door. Some have been in place for thousands of years. But there are other doors that you can kick open. By that, we must open our minds to different cultures and races. Why settle for white? What is wrong with a fellow Asian, Black, or Hispanic guy? If we restrict ourselves to Gay White Men, we, as Gay Asian Men, will continue to perpetuate stereotypes, and our self-esteem will take a beating. But that is easier said than done. It is rare to find gay Asian men who love Asians, Blacks, Latinos, or vice versa. As I mentioned earlier, all those races are chasing after the same thing—a white guy.

It is my hope for this essay and others I've written—for minds to change. I'm not suggesting that white guys shouldn't be with Asians. Nor am I saying that Asians shouldn't date older white men. If you, as a gay Asian man, find genuine attraction in an older man, I commend your choice. I assert that gay white men, in particular, view Asian men as undesirable in the gay community—period. Because the gay population is 90% white, we Asians don't stand a chance of breaking into that circle. The sooner we, as gay Asians, accept that, the happier we will be.

However, how can Asians accept knowing they are unwanted and invisible in the gay community? It is not easy. First, we must accept ourselves as beautiful people, no matter how many white guys reject us. After experiencing so many rejections, you may question your own qualities and shortcomings. I'm here to say nothing is wrong with you. You are a wonderful person, and you are fabulous. Don't feel depressed or inadequate about yourself because the latest white guy rejected you. It has nothing to do with you. You have done nothing wrong. The only problem is that you are not white.

Rejection from a white guy is not a catastrophic event. Enjoy your friends, hobbies, career, and sex when possible. This is my mantra when it comes to relationships. If it's destiny, it will find its way to me. Have an enjoyable and complete life without a boyfriend. Be patient; Mr. Right, regardless of age or race, will find you unexpectedly. Keep in mind that, despite facing ten thousand rejections, you will find someone.

After reading this essay, I hope some minds will change. That is all I wanted to do. For myself, I plan on being comfortable alone and waiting for a guy, regardless of race. I hope other gay Asian men read this and look beyond a person's ethnicity. You should fall in love with the person, not their skin color.

CHAPTER 4
The Gay Bathhouse Lunch Special

Do you mean that you've never heard of the lunch special, the one costing $8.00? When I told my friend, he exclaimed, "Wow, where can I get lunch that cheap?" Well, men are hungry. But it is not the food they are craving. At that hour, men are looking for quickie sex.

Most bathhouses (including the one I go to) feature a special lunch-hour rate, Monday through Friday. From 11:30 AM to 1:30 PM, a gay man can cruise a bathhouse for only $8.00. On a typical day, the noon crowd will have businessmen, bike couriers, students, delivery men, mail carriers, stay-at-home dads, and cab drivers. At that hour, you can find every profession represented. I often think the baths could host a career seminar at noon—like a "Lunch and Learn"!

It would take me roughly half an hour by bus to travel from my workplace to the bathhouse. As a result, I cannot make baths a regular part of my day. But I do have days off, so I dropped by at lunchtime out of curiosity. You first notice the number of parked cars outside the baths. Just outside the building, there are so many different types of automobiles. You have BMWs, Volvos, Station Wagons, Taxis, and every delivery truck from UPS to Pepsi lined up in a neat row. Students and couriers take their "lunch break" at the baths, stacking the bike rack outside. Cab drivers can accomplish two tasks simultaneously. After an hour of cruising and getting a quick fix at the baths, some cabbies will leave the bathhouse and wait for a fare. Some executives are always in a hurry to return to work.

Inside the bathhouse, there is a certain familiarity. Many of these men have seen each other daily at the gay bathhouse lunch hour. You can't help but overhear several different conversations at the same time. However, other lunchtime regulars do not initiate conversation, as they focus more on cruising to get laid. Some specifically seek out oral sex.

Many wives, girlfriends, and even fiancées don't like giving blowjobs, as they find it gross. What should a man do if he doesn't receive blowjobs at home? They go to the baths. Many straight men don't view oral sex as cheating or sex. They see it as a way to get off.

Regardless of the sexual orientation of these fully dressed businessmen, they all have one thing in common. These men only want a quick blowjob before heading back to the office. By remaining dressed, with the exception of an open zipper, these men indicate their desire for oral sex. These businessmen get what they want within ten minutes. That is the ultimate quickie. Let's face it, $8.00 is cheaper than getting a prostitute to do the deed!

During lunch hour, not just businesspeople and students frequent the gay baths. Many gay men who rely on disability checks for income also visit the baths at noon. Being on "disability" can cover every disease, from living with chronic pain to severe depression. Due to the limited coverage of a disability check, engaging in social activities with other gay men can be costly. The lunchtime special at the baths is the exception. Although rates vary from sauna to sauna, the noon-hour special at my local bathhouse is $8.00. For that price, men on disability can escape from their problems for six hours, albeit temporarily. They can cruise, indulge in eye candy, and engage in sexual activities like everyone else.

Being on disability might sound like a fabulous permanent vacation. But trust me, it gets boring after a while. Throughout your entire life, your focus has been either on school or your career. Qualifying for disability benefits relieves you of a significant burden. However, you quickly come to the realization that the world is slipping away from you. Men with disabilities must find other ways to occupy their time since most of their friends work. As a result, the baths become a central part of their lives. The baths instill a sense of purpose in these disabled men. Most disabled men use the baths at the beginning or end of the month. Why? That's when their check arrives in the mail.

As I observed all this, I wound up in the steam room next to another lunchtime regular. This guy works for the city, which has offices within walking distance of the Bathhouse. We talked for a few minutes, and I discovered why he goes to the baths daily at noon.

- It is $8.00, cheaper than lunch in the cafeteria.

- Getting off in the middle of the day is a fabulous stress reliever.

- It is a wonderful way to interact with some gay men in the middle of the day, especially when surrounded by straight co-workers from morning to afternoon.

As I continued my walk around the hallways, I noticed that certain men liked to advertise their occupations. A bike courier, passing by one room, hung his bike gear (including the wheel) on the wall as a visual display. Delivery men would be walking around wearing only a towel. The only difference was the company cap they wore. The day I was there, I saw hats that said "Pepsi" and "UPS."

As I left, I wistfully felt disappointed that I worked far away from the baths. The cost of lunch was $8.00. Where can you get a better bargain? If you have a job near a bathhouse, you should drop by for lunch one day. You never know who you might encounter.

Perhaps that adorable guy in accounting?

CHAPTER 5
Gay Quickies

One thing synonymous with a bathhouse is quickie sex, which takes place on an hourly basis. You would think that gay men would want to spend as much time as possible enjoying sex. However, many guys have told me that they prefer quickies because they are exactly that: They are concise and direct. There is no intimacy, no getting to know the other person, or any type of emotional bonding. Guys would rather save those feelings of pure lovemaking for someone they genuinely like.

That is one of the reasons why many men do not purchase a room when they visit the baths. Getting a room means subconsciously preparing for the possibility of spending quality time with another person. By getting a locker, you are categorizing sex as frequent and easy, with little hassle. You exchange no contact information, don't know each other's names, and don't need to show courtesy. You view each other as objects with the sole purpose of enjoying each other's bodies. Getting a locker also gives you an "out." Without a room, guys have no choice but to hook up openly. Because of that, it is easier to walk away from a sexual interlude that goes nowhere. If the same thing happens with two guys in a room, it is harder to kick someone out without being blunt or rude.

That's how the baths operate: they involve quick, straightforward sex.

Many men have told me that they even refrain from kissing other guys. Oral sex—no problem. Anal: pass the lube. But kissing? **NO WAY!** You would think it would be the other way around. I have always equated oral sex as a personal, intimate bonding experience between two people who genuinely care for one another. It's the opportunity to let go and give yourself to the other person. However, I must remove myself from the heterosexual perspective. In the homosexual world, the situation is reversed. In the gay world, kissing is equivalent to displaying intimate affection— between two guys who genuinely love each other. Whether it's oral or anal, you can experience it around the clock. Men want to save their actual, physical, close contact for a future boyfriend.

However, let us face reality. Because finding a partner or boyfriend is complex, many guys remain single for years between relationships. How many gay couples do you know that have lasted over a year? Therefore, quickie sex becomes a way to escape from that never-ending quest to find Mr. Right. That's why baths are the perfect place to satisfy your sexual craving fast. You save so much time at the baths compared to trolling through a hookup app. Scrolling through an online list of available guys is equivalent to the time it takes to arrive at the baths, get laid, and then return home.

Many guys are just looking for a quick blowjob or anal. They don't care about the location of the sex as long as it's brief and direct. I recall a businessman who arrived immaculately dressed. He stripped off his clothes, went to someone's room, took a shower, got dressed, and then left. This entire process took only 20 minutes! You would think that when a man enters the baths with six hours to spare, he will spend all six hours with a guy he's just met. However, the issue lies in the intimacy factor. Men often avoid getting close to a guy unless there is a developing relationship. Gay men view the gay baths as a means to ejaculate until their next encounter.

That is what 's so great about the baths. Sex is easily accessible and direct. It is common for guys to have three to five quickies in an hour! Men can spend as little as ten minutes at the gay baths. However, diversity is indeed the essence of life. Having sex out in the open is bound to attract a crowd. However, if you see two men going at it in public,

Can you stay and watch?

Can you join them?

Just what is the etiquette?

Here's the etiquette to watch and join in.

What is the protocol to observe? How do you handle it? If I am in the sauna or steam room and two guys suddenly come in and start making out, I can stay and watch. I arrived first, so if they had a problem, they wouldn't have come in. However, if the couple had entered the sauna or steam room before me and began engaging in sexual activities, I would refrain from entering and would stay away. You don't know how comfortable they are with people watching. Most of the time, men find it uncomfortable when others watch them engage in sexual activity. If a couple feels like too many eyes are watching, they will leave to find a private area.

Regrettably, certain individuals at the baths will follow a couple who are attempting to have a quickie. These men will follow the couple from room to room, wanting to "watch." That is poor bathhouse etiquette. However, some couples are pure exhibitionists, having no problem with an audience. Therefore, if a crowd watches two guys going at it, you can observe. Let's face it: This is a live sex show, complete with full-on hard-ons. How often do you see that? Porn movies notwithstanding.

But could you join in and make it a threesome instead of watching? It does happen that other men will join in, making it a threesome or even a foursome. But what is the etiquette for joining in? It depends on the situation. If you see two guys getting it on, wait for a signal from them that you can participate. A wink, a nod, or even a hand wave will give you an indication. If you don't see any of these signs, they may be uninterested in a third party. If you attempt to join in without a sign, you may face pushback. This can happen either gently or with great force. That is embarrassing, so wait for the signals. If you do not care about being shot down, go for it. However, be aware that physical pushing may serve as a warning to retreat. Again, you cannot take this rejection personally; that is how the baths are.

Now that you understand the proper etiquette for witnessing and participating in group sex, let's explore the areas in a bathhouse where these intimate moments can take place: The wet area, which includes the sauna, steam, whirlpool, and shower; the porn lounge; and lastly, the orgy room are the areas where these quickies can transpire in a bathhouse.

The Wet Area

It's an area where men eventually converge during their travels inside a bathhouse. This section usually has showers, a whirlpool, a sauna or steam room, a sink and mirrors, and a toilet. Men often congregate in the wet area, cruising and seeking their next sexual encounter. Eventually, many guys cruising a bathhouse's hallways will wind up in the sauna or steam room.

Sauna or Steam Room

Quickie encounters between two guys in the sauna will happen one of two ways. By chance, two men end up there. Alternatively, one individual pursues the other into the sauna. As the two men sit together in the sauna, they establish eye contact to gauge any potential interest.

If there is interest, one of the men will start to stroke until he achieves a full erection. If the other guy is not interested, he will leave. But if he stays, the next step is to touch each other's erections. Finally, they suck each other off. These quickies in a sauna usually last ten to fifteen minutes. Because of the heat inside the sauna, fresh air is necessary to breathe, so these sauna quickies don't last long. Couples must leave the steam to continue their liaison elsewhere in the baths. But some guys have incredible staying power, going on for over an hour in the heat!

Whirlpool

A quickie in a whirlpool presents its own unique set of circumstances. I have a friend named Mike who visits the bathhouse strictly for relaxation. I don't think he cares if he gets off, as Mike spends almost all his time in the pool. But what if a charming guy dips in? Mike will make the first move. First, he positions himself, so he is opposite or near the guy. Then Mike "accidentally" brushes his leg against the other guy. If he does not respond or moves away, then Mike knows the other guy is uninterested. But if the guy returns the "accidental brush" with his own feet, then Mike starts to reel him in. Initially, Mike engages in footsies with the other man, raising his foot to a level where he can massage the other guy's genitalia. These two guys will soon feel each other up with some oral and simulating anal—all within a 15-minute encounter in the whirlpool. Most likely, an audience will gather to observe this whirlpool encounter. Due to the intense heat, the man will likely exit the whirlpool and walk away. Neither man has ejaculated. Mike usually stays in the pool, relaxing and enjoying the waves. Mike is satisfied for the time being, until the next guy enters the whirlpool.

Shower Area

The baths' shower areas are popular for quickie sex. Similar to the sauna area, guys enjoy cruising each other while taking a shower. In an effort to attract attention, guys will start off by soaping up their cock until achieving a full erection. Some men skip soaping up their dick in order to be more direct. Reaching out to touch the other guy's cock is another tactic. If the other guy is uninterested, he will say, "No thanks," and walk away. But if the other guy is interested, he will reciprocate. Soon the two guys begin caressing and soaping each other, sliding their wet, soapy bodies together. Soon, one of the guys will start sucking the other guy off. Both showerheads are still running full blast, with steaming hot water falling on both men.

Guys hook up in the wet area more often than you might think. Couples face a problem with how open the wet area is. There is no privacy, so naturally, couples leave the wet area to escape the stares and crowds. Unfortunately, if neither man has a room, they have one of three choices. First, one of the guys can exchange their locker for a room. Secondly, they can both change into new clothes and inquire, "Your place or mine?" Third, they can find a more discreet place in the bathhouse, usually the porn lounge or the orgy room. Both of those rooms are where most quickies typically take place.

Porn Lounge

The porn lounge is sort of like the sauna. It is the one room where I have seen the wildest action. Over the years, I have seen my share of rimming, oral, threesomes, and foursomes in the porn lounge. The main difference between the sauna and the porn lounge is that you can see gay porn images onscreen. Simultaneously, you can witness men stroking themselves to ejaculate as they watch gay porn. The porn lounge is the one area of the baths that elicits the quickest sex. Like in a sauna, if two guys find each other hot while stroking themselves to full erections, they will go for it. In front of an audience, they engage in kissing, suckling, and rimming each other with fully erect cocks. Oftentimes, having so many people watching them can make a couple feel uncomfortable. So, they put a chair in front of them (as if that would help). Most times, a couple leaves to find a dark corner in a hallway or even an unoccupied restroom stall.

At one point, I entered the porn lounge and was taken aback by the sight of two men engaging in raw anal sex. The two men assumed the following positions: Guy A was sitting, and Guy B was sitting on him, pumping up and down. After a few minutes, Guy A grabbed Guy B, lifted him, positioned him on all fours (doggy style), and started to pump him again, thrusting his cock in and out. After another few minutes, they changed positions; Guy B was lying on his back, with Guy A continuing to pump his cock in and out. After another few minutes, Guy B got up, leaned against the wall, and had Guy A pump him out of that position. After that, they seemed worn out and stopped. Neither man came, nor were condoms used. They chitchatted for a bit, with Guy A saying he could go for hours without ejaculating. Guy B expressed his gratitude and continued his journey.

Dark Room

The last place you can get quickie sex in a bathhouse is the darkroom (or the orgy room). This room also serves couples looking for privacy (when both parties only have a locker).

Many couples enjoy having sex openly in a dark room, on a bench, or in slings. They relish having men stare at them while having sex. These are the guys who like to be voyeurs.

The darkness envelopes you as soon as you enter the darkroom. You can hardly make out what other guys are doing. So, you have to wait for your eyes to adjust to the darkness. But once your eyes change, you see shadows and bodies moving, giving couples some privacy. Most times you stand there and watch others have sex in the darkness.

These rooms can feature everything from open booths (like a telephone booth so you can have privacy), multiple Glory Holes for group play, and other dark (or pitch-dark) spaces with some benches (in case two guys want to do anal).

Years ago, an episode of "Queer as Folk" showed an orgy room inside a bathhouse. When that episode hit the airwaves, I received dozens of requests from men asking me to recommend a bathhouse in their city. The scenes featured dozens of men all having sex with one another, oblivious to who was watching. In my opinion, that scene is pure fiction. In the twenty-plus years that I have gone to the baths, I have never seen multiple orgies. I might have seen a foursome once or twice, but that was it. I say it is fiction because group sex is supposed to be an unbridled passion where guys just go for it, regardless of the other person's appearance.

In theory, that is what group sex should be. However, gay men have preferences. For group sex to be successful, everyone in the group must feel attracted to each other. That doesn't happen. It is possible for one person to find only certain individuals attractive. Simultaneously, someone else might find only one individual attractive. So instead of this big 20-person session, you have different groups of three or four going at it. You may switch between groups, but in reality, it is five separate groups rather than a single group of 20. For one big sex group to function, all 20 people must find each other attractive. It's impossible to arrange a spontaneous 20-person sex session at the baths without prior planning. When group sex occurs in these dark rooms, it signifies a desperation for sexual activity that compels all participants to blindly pursue unknown individuals. However, if someone were to suddenly turn on the lights in a dark room during a 20-person group session, the session would immediately break up due to superficial bias.

With so many men available in a bathhouse for a 15-minute "quickie," you might ask yourself, "Where are the men who like to cuddle?" That's my favorite form of sex, just between you and me.

Please stay tuned for my next story, where I will demonstrate the concept of "Real Men Cuddle."

My second book, "Back To The Baths: More Gay Bathhouse Stories," features this story.

CHAPTER 6
Straight & Bi Married Men At The Baths

At the baths, watching men cruise each other for a hookup is enjoyable to observe. One of my favorite pastimes is sitting in one of the busiest hallways, seeing all the men pass me by, and focusing on their left hands. Why? I like to see how many wedding rings I can pick out. My record was to count 20 wedding rings in a single night. But since same-sex marriage is now legal, this little game I play no longer applies!

Married men can freely express themselves in the baths without fear of detection. As previously mentioned, a gay bathhouse provides a discreet environment. It is too risky for married men to go to a gay bar to hook up for sex for three reasons.

- One: Someone constantly worries about being "seen" by someone.

- Two: Engaging in conversation with someone at a bar takes too much time.

- Three: If married men find someone, they have nowhere to go to have sex.

The baths are incredibly convenient, providing a direct and efficient experience. You are in a convenient location with a room just around the corner, allowing you to quickly hook up. But many married men go to the baths, looking for some companionship in a non-sexual way. These men don't have many dealings with the gay community, and the need to connect with other gay men is strong. Whether they're engaging in a conversation or witnessing two men enjoying a quickie, it satisfies their desire to interact with other men. Closeted men feel safer connecting with other gay men at the baths because it is private, much more so than a bar or club. What bathhouses offer is a false sense of security and acceptance. This feeling of liberation allows one to release their inhibitions and feel unrestrained.

But it's not just married men who use the baths to fool around. I've interacted with many gay men in committed relationships that are not open. An interesting fact: some of these men can't ejaculate despite being turned on. The reason? If they come earlier in the day with someone else at a bathhouse and then cannot come later that same day with their significant other, suspicion will arise. But that is only for gay men. Married men are more relaxed, as they do not have to worry about ejaculation. They can complain to their wife about a headache.

Typically, married men go to the baths during the day, never late at night when it's the busiest. You can catch married men at the baths three different times: during lunchtime, after work, and on Sunday afternoons when football is on TV. In a previous chapter entitled "The Lunch Special," I've already written about the lunchtime crowd. The after-work crowd consists of commuters who want to wait out the rush hour. With nothing to do from 5 PM to 8 PM, these men will head to the baths looking for some action. Typically, they inform their wives that they have a client meeting, are working late at the office, or are stuck in heavy traffic. The Sunday afternoon crowd consists of other married men looking for hot sex before dinner with the folks. Excuses for their wives range from having to finish up some work at the office, going to the gym, or having a beer with their buddies at a bar while watching football.

I have met and seen my share of married men at the baths over the years; here is one example. Imagine a bodybuilder with a model's face and hair. He wears torn jeans and a sleeveless flannel shirt. But he is married, lives in the closet, and visits the gay baths on a weekly basis. I once overheard a conversation he had with another guy. They had just finished having sex. He told the other man he'd be first in line for a pill to make him straight. It made me think about what his life would be like if he were honest with himself. He would not be alone; he would be extremely popular in the gay community. However, he is married and remains in the closet. If I were to encounter him on the street, I would perceive him as straight.

Then there are the married and single straight men who use the baths to get a blowjob. Many women dislike performing orally for their husbands, boyfriends, or partners. They find it gross and prefer the conventional way of sex. When their partner denies oral sex, these men feel they must visit the baths for a blow job. The guy performing oral doesn't have to look great. All that straight guy is concentrating on is the fabulous feeling of getting blown. Numerous straight men can be observed in the porn room, stroking their cocks as they sit with an erection. Eventually, other men will come crawling. I recall a man who took pleasure solely in receiving oral sex. Every week, he would arrive at the baths on the same day and time. He would plunk himself in the porn room, stroke himself, and soon more than twenty guys would suck him for over three hours! During that time, he would say nothing. Some blowjobs lasted 60 seconds; others could go on for twenty minutes. After three hours, he would shower and leave. This pattern would repeat itself every seven days. Guys used to wait by the porn room for him because he proved to be so popular and consistent.

Other married men I've seen at the baths arrive with hustlers they have a relationship with. Each week, they gather at the baths, engage in passionate sexual activities, and then part ways. After another seven days, they reunite. As I mentioned in my essay, Tricks of the Trade, a trick is not a one-night stand in a hustler's mind. A successful "trick" is when you get a customer returning for more and more; that way, a hustler has a guaranteed income source.

Then there are the older married men who have been cruising the bathhouse hallways for decades. In the 1950s and early 1960s, men were marrying women. That was the thing to do. Many of them believed that getting married would eliminate their feelings for men. Now decades later, they accept their sexuality but lack the courage to break up the family. It can be challenging when a situation remains unchanged for more than two decades. However, surprisingly, I have met some older married men who have come out to their wives and now have a marriage in name only. Not wanting to break up the family, both the husband and wife pursue new relationships outside the marriage. But I have also met some other married men who have since divorced their wives. They did not want to live a lie any longer, and I salute their courage. It's challenging to come out at 50 or 60 today. While gay acceptance is growing, older gay people are more invisible in the gay community, which emphasizes youth and beauty.

To sum it up, why do married men go to the baths? Half of them are in denial about their sexuality. Despite vowing never to revisit the Baths, these men keep coming back. The other half accepts their sexuality and returns to the baths for companionship. They are perpetually concerned about their current spouse discovering the truth.

I hope all these married men practice safe sex—for their wives' sake.

CHAPTER 7
Accessories

You would think the only thing coming between you and a hot guy at the baths would be the towels both of you are wearing. However, you will often see guys wearing more than just their towels to get extra attention, known as accessorizing. At the baths, you want to impress other guys with your accessories. Standing out amongst the crowd sends a specific signal to other guys. Conversely, you might choose to accessorize for comfort. Whatever the reason, if you regularly visit the baths, it is always beneficial to come prepared with a few items. Here are the most common things men bring with them.

Leather

Some men like to enhance their towel appearance by adding leather. Over the years, I have seen various men in leather at the baths. But overwhelmingly, most men wearing leather at the tubs are BEARS. Wearing leather is a strong signal to other guys interested in S&M or any other type of dominance. The message conveys that you share their interest in similar activities. The fashion statement of wearing leather at the baths varies between men. Some wear a leather vest with a towel. Others have leather straps over their chests and arms. Some individuals choose to wear a leather hat. However, some men will wear a leather strap over just one arm. This is done to communicate their preferences to other men. The strap on the left means top, or dominant. At the same time, a strap on the right implies bottom or submissive. Straps on both arms mean they can be versatile.

However, a few guys disregard the towel and wear a fetish leather outfit with leather pants, a hat, and boots. Notable is the number of leather cock rings worn, particularly by men over sixty. Wearing a cock ring supposedly keeps an erection up for a long time, even after ejaculation. Every time I visit the baths; I see many elderly gay men wearing them. I would have thought Viagra was supposed to put the cock ring industry out of business!

Footwear

Many guys are very paranoid about what their naked feet may step on. Bathhouses are so dark, you can't see what's on the floor. That is especially true in bathrooms, where some baths do not have urinals. The toilet area often appears "wet." Semen may be present on the floor of the porn lounge or any other central cruising location where men engage in sexual activity. So many guys don various footwear—sandals, flip-flops, bedroom slippers, and even socks—as they cruise up and down the hallways. I do not recommend wearing socks because your feet will get wet and uncomfortable if you pass through the "wet" area. Generally speaking, much older men (in their early sixties) and Asian men (due to paranoia) usually wear footwear at the baths. I've even observed some Asian men wearing both socks and sneakers. That is real paranoia, and it just looks silly. Wearing sandals has crossed my mind, but I have decided against it. I think wearing something on your feet defeats the feeling of total nakedness at the baths. I love that feeling, and wearing footwear does not make me feel the same.

Underwear

Some men will be at the baths naked, with a towel on, but wearing a t-shirt. That signifies the man's insecurity about his "physique." You might think that he is feeling cold. No. In the winter, management usually raises the temperature to summer-like levels. Since 99% of the gay population is obsessed with body image, many guys feel apprehensive about showing their merchandise. Gay men worry it may hurt their chances of hooking up with someone. It can seem competitive and threatening at the baths, surrounded by Twinks with 5% body fat. Because of that, some gay men tend to cover up what makes them insecure. Gay men often wear a baseball cap to hide their thinning hair. If their stomach is visible, they cover it with a shirt.

But not everyone is insecure. You have the gym bunnies, who enjoy visiting the baths to showcase their bodies. They don't wear a towel but instead wear their designer underwear. They strut up and down the hallways, as if walking the runways of a fashion show.

You may see a guy now and then at the baths wearing nothing. That is right—completely nude as he cruises the hallways. Rules state that everyone has to wear something to cover their midsection. But management does not try to enforce that rule. Once in a while, a bathhouse staff person tells the "nudist" to wear a towel, but that is rare. Being naked does have its drawbacks. Now that everyone has seen the merchandise, the mystery surrounding the man is no longer present. Based on what they have seen, some guys may take a pass. If the male merchandise is unbelievable, advertising may be beneficial in attracting attention.

People frequently inquire about whether it's possible to attend the baths solely as an observer without encountering unwanted attention. The answer is yes, and here's the secret. Do not get undressed. No rule says you have to take off all of your clothes. Being fully dressed is a sign to other guys that you are off-limits. Some men might even think you work at the bathhouse, as all patrons know that staff is off-limits. My friend Ari will do just that. When he goes to the baths, he stays fully clothed, sits in a part of the bathhouse, and watches people passing him by. No one bothers him. If he sees someone attractive, he will pursue him while fully clothed.

Handheld Items

While cruising the halls looking for the next hookup, many guys carry stuff to occupy themselves during the down periods at the baths. Men frequently carry items like water bottles for hydration, cigarettes for smoking, condoms and lube for preparation, and books for entertainment. Some guys even carry their cell phones with them—a practice I strongly discourage due to the high risk of theft or misplacing them. So many guys have lost their room or locker keys over the years. Having your cell phone vanish would be an even more irreplaceable item. I would advise you to keep any expensive valuables in your car. Some gay bathhouses will allow you to keep your personal effects in a separate safe, monitored by the desk clerk. But by far, the most popular item men carry with them at the baths is Amyl Nitrate, better known as "poppers." This drug is prevalent in the gay community, as it enhances the intensity of an orgasm and relaxes the anal area during sex. You can understand why men adore their poppers and refuse to leave home without them. Some men wear a small bottle of poppers on a chain around their neck so it is readily available. You need to be ready for the influx of quickies at any given time. I see more men carrying around poppers than condoms!

Toiletries

Showering between each sexual encounter is beneficial. This ensures that you arrive at your next hookup feeling refreshed. All bathhouses have liquid soap in the shower area, but it can be harsh and dry for your skin. It is common for many guys to bring their own personal toiletry items. You see them carrying a small bag with soap, shampoo, hair gel, a shaving kit, aftershave, deodorant, and moisturizer. Being in a bathhouse without the necessary toiletries is the worst experience. A quick trip to the drugstore is impossible. You cannot leave the gay baths for any reason without losing your room or locker (this is to avoid drug trafficking on the premises). Only those customers from out of town can purchase in-and-out privileges, but even then they must provide ID to prove they are from out of state. So, it is beneficial to come prepared with everything you may need.

Items for the Nightstand

Every room at the baths has a nightstand beside the bed where you can put your cigarettes, water bottles, and other assorted items. When cruising the hallways and passing dozens of rooms, the one constant you will see is condoms and lube on the nightstand. Sometimes, you may even see poppers! Having lubricant and condoms visible next to the bed sends a signal to other guys interested in anal sex. But it can work the opposite way. Some guys who are not interested in anal sex or barebacking will avoid rooms containing condoms.

Some men prepare for everything. I know a man who goes to great lengths in his preparation. Every time he visits the baths, he comes prepared. The nightstand is overflowing with stuff. There are condoms, two different brands of lube, moisturizer, massage oil, a box of Kleenex, a roll of paper towels, water, a package of wipes, scented candles, a small clock, a little radio (for jazz music), shampoo, liquid soap, hair gel, poppers, and a pack of cigarettes. This guy doesn't even inhale poppers or smoke cigarettes. But he brings them anyway for any potential 'hookups' with men who may require these items during their romantic encounter. Isn't that so thoughtful?

These are just a few of the item's men bring with them to the gay baths. Most gay bathhouse visits are impulsive, so keep some of the stuff I've mentioned in your car. That way, you can be prepared, making your next visit to the baths all the more pleasurable.

CHAPTER 8
Tricks of the Trade

The minute I saw him; I knew his motives. He had blond hair, blue eyes, and a gorgeous physique. I would assume he is in his mid-twenties. He was not completely naked, unlike the rest of us cruising through the baths. However, he was shirtless, wearing his pants just loose enough to show the top of his briefs. So, what type of guy do you think I am describing? If you said hustler, you'd be right. He was semi-dressed, which was the giveaway. If he were a regular customer, he would have stripped off his clothes like the rest of us. Because he wasn't wearing a towel, the hustler didn't feel inclined to engage in sexual activities, as this is a job, not a place for pleasure.

Regular bathhouse visitors will eventually come across a hustler. There's nothing a bathhouse can do to stop it. After all, it is the oldest profession in history. I once went to a bathhouse in another state. Upon entering, I immediately noticed a sign prohibiting solicitation. Thirty minutes later, a hustler propositioned me for an $85 experience. How can you identify when someone is attempting to proposition you? Here's an easy way to find out: Suppose an Abercrombie and Fitch type approaches you and starts to make conversation. He is a hustler. Individual Abercrombie and Fitch types who are not hustlers tend to attract others who are similar to them. If you don't fit that stereotype and someone similar approaches you to initiate a conversation, I can assure you that their intention is to make quick cash.

The blond guy sized me up and approached me with a friendly hello. We eventually ended up in the lounge, talking. That is the first move a hustler will make. Experienced hustlers know which men to target: Asians and older gay men. These two groups of men struggle to find sex. After spending hours observing naked bodies walking around in the lounge and watching pornographic movies, these men desperately crave sex. The hustler enters the scene, knowing that these men are desperate for sex. So they start a conversation, saying they are selling their bodies. They dangle their sexuality in front of these men, to the point where they cannot refuse.

The blonde guy and I exchanged names, with Stephen being his. I ask him if he is gay, and he tells me yes. I look at Stephen and try to visualize his life before he wound up hustling on the streets. He looked like the typical homogeneous suburban twink. In high school, he probably was well-liked, athletic, and a popular choice among women. What could go wrong? Perhaps his parents kicked him out for being gay? It is possible. The sexual orientation of a hustler is 50/50. The majority survive by hustling on the streets. Having left broken homes, these guys wind up on the streets. These individuals are willing to go to extreme measures to earn a living, frequently turning to substances such as crack or heroin to alleviate their emotional distress. Eventually, an addiction develops. These twinks now hustle not to eat but to keep their habit alive.

Stephen and I continued to chitchat when he finally got around to telling me that he was "working." At the baths, you will encounter two types of hustlers. The first type advertises themselves as "masseuses." They'll go up to men and ask if they want a massage. Generally, a masseuse will charge 70 to 100 dollars for a rubdown. Unfortunately, most of these hustlers who pitch themselves as masseuses are inept.

They move their hands over your body, not getting into the muscles. But all of these masseuses have one goal in mind. The goal is to arouse the customer's sexual desire. That is when extras are offered. Typically, a handjob is an extra $50, oral $75, sexual relations (kissing, sucking) $75, and full-fledged anal $200. These extras are in addition to the massage, which could net someone over $300 for an hour's work. For years, some men have dedicated themselves to the "masseuse" profession, eschewing the allure of drugs or prostitution. This is the career they have chosen. Some are still plugging away in their mid-forties, with a full slate of regular customers.

Similar to a masseuse, the other type of hustler focuses on providing a range of prices. The trick here is for the hustler to spend as little time as possible. If you agree on half an hour, the hustler will typically perform for only 20 minutes. The customer is unaware of the scam; he has just experienced oral sex and feels elated. These hustlers get hardened fast. To them, a trick is more than just a one-time deal. When you get a customer to return for more, it's an excellent trick. That way, a hustler has a guaranteed source of income for a while, at least until they can secure another customer. A friend of mine was caught in this trap.

Years ago, my friend once served as a sugar daddy for a hustler. It occurred during a time in his life when he had no self-esteem. This hustler was his addiction, and my friend kept returning for more. The amount of money he lavished on this hustler was beyond his comprehension. My friend thought they had a relationship. But now he knows better; the hustler was just there for the money—to support his massive heroin addiction. Be aware that these hustlers want to extort as much money as possible out of the customer. Just because a hustler may appear friendly, that does not mean they won't screw someone over for a buck.

Regarding my friend's trick, he expresses relief for never exchanging personal information. They initially met at the baths and kept everything in that environment. Afterwards, my friend discovered that his hustler was serving a prison sentence for drug-related offenses. Therefore, he considers himself fortunate to have parted ways with him.

Stephen strikes me as a typical hustler. They all act the same. Once they gain someone's sympathy, they understand they have a chance to earn money. Stephen is no exception. Stephen begins to narrate a heartbreaking tale about his homelessness, lack of financial resources, and lack of a place to reside. Feeling sympathy for Stephen, I gave him $10.00 to renew his locker and a coupon for a free room for a future visit, without any conditions. He asks why I do not want to sleep with him.

There is no shame in hiring a sex worker. Why not pursue the opportunity if the sole obstacle between you and a desirable individual is a mere $100? But here is the problem: a majority of hustlers have no passion. For them, this is work. It is not sex that is enjoyable. Some men have no self-esteem, making them an effortless mark for many hustlers. You should be confident enough to know that sex should not cost you.

Many of the hustlers are straight. One gay-for-pay hustler told me that what drives him during sex is not sexual gratification but the amount of money he will make once the sex is over. The ultimate goal is to get a profitable trick, so they keep returning for more, thus regularly filling the hustler's wallet. Another straight hustler I know has been hustling for the past ten years. He began his hustle by taking on the next-door neighbor, and it quickly escalated to the point where he now engages in it occasionally to earn extra money. Whenever he is between jobs and has no money, he picks himself up and heads to the baths to seek a score. He even has some regular customers. I once asked him how he could do that. How was he able to be with a guy and have sex with him without feeling any physical attraction? You do what you have to do to survive, he told me. So, he will suck, kiss, and cuddle. However, he refuses to engage in anal sex. Additionally, he is selective about the guys he chooses. He sets boundaries with overweight or elderly people. But as I mentioned, these hustlers (most of whom are straight) have a drug habit to support. Hustling is their sole source of income, which explains their motivation, even in the face of zero attraction from their customers.

While some hustlers exhibit a work ethic akin to those I've described, others are like rag dolls. They lie there, expecting the customer to do all of the work. You may need to explicitly tell the hustler what to do in bed, since they are often robotic and repeat tasks. So, if you are passive, hiring a hustler at the baths might be a waste of money, depending on the sex worker you hire. If you are aggressive in bed, you will receive value for your money.

Then you get into the sticky situation of running into that hustler again at the baths. Remember what I wrote earlier? Hustlers search for regular customers so they have a consistent income. It is awkward to turn someone down who is desperate for cash. My recommendation is to explain that you didn't anticipate their presence and are experiencing financial difficulties.

Returning to Stephen, he pulls out his pipe and takes a puff of crack. In between his inhalations, I learned a bit more about him. I discovered he has been hustling for about ten years (he is 30 now). He hails from a broken family, lacks prospects outside of hustling, and recently received his release from jail for assault. His lean, muscular body is a result of his prison time. There was nothing else to do other than lift weights. I shudder to think about what type of sex he had or if he injected heroin in prison. I would not be surprised if he had HIV.

We talk for a bit longer, and then we exit my room. As I head to hit the showers, Stephen makes a detour to the locker area. He's checking out the gay baths because he wants to score more crack cocaine. As he heads out, he says, "The way I am going, death is just around the corner." And you know what? I believe him.

CHAPTER 9
Drug Use At The Gay Baths Part 1

The following is a true story. The customer in Room 3-1-6 was late—on real overtime! He checked in around 8 PM the previous night, and now noon was approaching, just in time for the lunch special. Generally, there is a grace period for customers who run overtime for an hour or so. However, the occupant of Room 3-1-6 had been in that room for 16 hours, four of which were overtime, as he rented a 12-hour room. The desk attendant repeatedly announced via the loudspeaker that Room 3-1-6 was on overtime. So, he should either check out or renew. For hours, there was no response to the frequent calls to check out, only silence from the floor attendant's repeated knocking on the door.

Finally, the floor attendant decided it was time to burst in and wake up the delinquent customer. It's not uncommon for customers to stay late for extended periods. The occupant of Room 3-1-6 was probably still sleeping off his hangover from the previous night's partying. Having a 12-hour room provides customers with in-and-out privileges. He could have gone barhopping before returning to the baths to crash. The floor attendant knocked a final time, announcing it was time to check out or renew. Hearing no response, the floor attendant inserted his master key and tried to open the door. But it would not open. Thinking it was a jammed door, the floor attendant started pushing and, to his horror, realized that wasn't the case. The customer lay dead, slumped against the door. The autopsy report later stated that the death happened around 10:00 PM. The customer lay lifeless in his room for a duration of 14 hours. Considering he was found against a closed door; it seems like the customer was making a feeble attempt to save himself. Numerous men engaged in sexual activity in the rooms surrounding him, leaving the customer to die in silence.

This little vignette illustrates the reckless drug use prevalent in the gay community. Using illegal substances seems to be a part of mainstream gay culture. It is as common as having that cup of coffee in the morning. As a gay man, you see drugs taken at clubs, bars, and private parties. So why should anyone be surprised that drugs are rampant in a bathhouse? To their credit, bathhouses generally prohibit the consumption of any recreational drugs used on the premises. Upon entering any American bathhouse, you will notice a sign stating, "We do not allow the use of alcohol and drugs." However, how can the staff effectively monitor activities taking place behind closed doors? Entering a bathhouse doesn't require a strip search. Gay saunas prioritize privacy, and we should respect that. In addition, half the staff uses drugs recreationally in their personal lives, so why should they judge someone else? But when a bathhouse has to call the paramedics every Saturday night (due to a possible overdose), you know there is a problem.

These two essays will provide a comprehensive analysis of the drug and alcohol scene at the baths, revealing a complex and unsettling reality. This world consists of drugs, alcohol, and mindless sex. Remember, gay baths are a fantasy world where gay men can do whatever they want. Within those walls, nothing is sacred.

Of all the drugs consumed at the gay baths, marijuana seems the least dangerous. Gay men consider it so minor that it is not unusual to witness customers and bathhouse staff sharing a joint. The scent of marijuana often hits you as soon as you walk in, as you can smell the odor from individual rooms, even walking down the halls. After a three- or four-hour marathon of sex, some couples will relax in the afterglow by sharing a joint. Some gay men even light up before heading to the baths. It helps to loosen them up so they do not feel inhibited. Therefore, they either use cannabis or take a few shots of alcohol to achieve the desired readiness for sex.

Rarely have I witnessed someone so inebriated in the baths that they crash into walls and furniture. Drunks at the gay baths are a business liability, as they will drive customers away. If someone shows up to be intoxicated and wants to get in, the desk attendant will likely turn them away. Many bathhouses lack liquor licenses, making alcohol consumption strictly prohibited. However, this does not prevent men from openly and discreetly consuming booze during their stay. You will not see guys holding a vodka bottle or beer while walking up and down the halls. Instead, they will be carrying plastic bottles containing alcohol disguised as soda. The plastic bottles are filled with transparent liquid, so you cannot tell if it is liquor. The customer's locker always contains more alcohol, allowing them to refill their empty soda bottle.

Most gay men who drink in the baths can hold their beer. Over the years, I've seen drunk men passed out. Alternatively, you may witness intoxicated men sitting in the lounge, speaking incoherently to anyone who will listen. Some gay saunas do have a liquor license and allow alcohol consumption. However, their liquor license only permits alcohol consumption in the bar area, not in private rooms.

Amyl nitrate, also known as poppers, is the most popular minor drug among gay men. It's a substance that increases sexual pleasure. Poppers are also known for their ability to increase the intensity of an orgasm and relax the anal area during sexual intercourse, which is particularly beneficial for exclusive bottoms. You can understand why men adore their poppers and refuse to leave home without them. Some men will even wear a small bottle of poppers on a chain around their neck, like a necklace. Given the prevalence of quickies at the baths, it's crucial to be prepared for unexpected encounters. I even see more men carrying around poppers than condoms! Poppers are technically illegal without a prescription. Nonetheless, many bathhouses and sex stores sell them. You can even buy them online by searching the word "poppers." However, when you mix poppers or other drugs, it can be a lethal cocktail. Poppers, combined with either Viagra or Crystal Meth, can drop blood pressure to dangerously low levels.

Now we get to the severe drugs consumed at the baths: Crystal Meth (with fentanyl mixed in), GHB, ecstasy, Special K, Speed, and Crack Cocaine. While men consume marijuana and poppers openly at the baths, they consume these hardcore drugs more discreetly. But let's return to Viagra for a moment and consider why this drug is so common in the club scene. After all, it is associated with older men, and these young twinks certainly do not need help in that department. But long-term use of Ecstasy (also known as "E") or Crystal Meth can cause erectile dysfunction. Taking Viagra solves that problem and actually intensifies its effects when combined with other party drugs. Ecstasy in combination with GHB (also known as "G") and Special K (also known as "K"). How do drug users distinguish between safe and unsafe combinations? Someone once told me that when using party drugs, you can mix a drug with a vowel (E) and a drug with consonants (G & K), but you shouldn't mix the consonant drugs (G & K) at all!

But by far, the most commonly used drug at the baths (other than poppers) is Crystal Meth. It is similar to Ecstasy (an amphetamine), as Crystal Meth is methamphetamine—hence the word "meth" in Crystal Meth. Ecstasy and Crystal Meth make you hyper and talkative, cause intense pleasure, and suppress appetite. But methamphetamines (crystal meth) are much more potent than amphetamines (ecstasy), which is why meth is so popular. In addition, meth can give men the body they have always wanted. How? As mentioned, meth suppresses one's appetite. Many young gay men who use meth become anorexic, with only 5% body fat.

If these gay men take GHB instead (remember, you **DO NOT** mix GHB with Meth), this drug allegedly stimulates growth hormones, acting as an anabolic steroid. Therefore, gay men can achieve a muscular physique without engaging in any physical activity. However, exercise is often the last thing on many people's minds. Their top priorities are club drugs, circuit parties, and party & play (also known as PNP). The irony about PNP is that taking all these drugs (like Crystal Meth) causes erectile dysfunction. Therefore, these drug users experience high levels of sexual arousal but have a limp cock. People even refer to this phenomenon as "Crystal Dick." Which causes most drug users to wind up being the recipients of anal sex in all these Chem Sex encounters, as they can't achieve an erection. However, PNP men often use Viagra in conjunction with Crystal Meth to achieve an erect cock, a practice that is not recommended.

We now turn our attention to the safety aspect of using party substances. I do not recommend doing drugs; in fact, I am **VERY ANTI-DRUG**. However, all the moralizing and finger-pointing won't deter gay men from using these substances. Therefore, gay men should educate themselves on what to do in the event that they or a drug associate overdoses. First, the following five signs indicate when someone is overdosing:

One: Shallow breathing

Two: Clammy and cool skin

Three: The inability to wake up or fall asleep.

Four: Small Pupils

Fifth: The body becomes limp.

If you are going to be doing drugs with someone, **ALWAYS** carry Naloxone with you, as those drugs might contain fentanyl. Naloxone is a tool that has the ability to rapidly save the life of someone who overdoses, as it counteracts the effects of opioids. This medication only works on opioid-related overdoses; it will do no harm if the overdose is non-opioid-related. If you plan to use Naloxone with someone else, ensure that both of you are familiar with its use. It is available either as an easy-to-use nasal spray, or you can inject it like an EpiPen, so anyone can administer it. If someone you are with has an overdose, it is important that you administer Naloxone and call 911 immediately, as the person needs medical attention no matter what. Do not be afraid to call for help. Most likely, authorities will not charge you with drug possession because they prioritize saving someone's life over busting someone for narcotics. Most jurisdictions have what is known as the "Good Samaritan Law," meaning that if a person does the right thing, they will be immune from prosecution. Since most pharmacies offer Naloxone without a prescription, there's no reason not to get it. If the pharmacy in your area does not provide this drug, you can obtain it from other organizations without any questions. However, it is up to you to seek out Naloxone for your own safety. Before using drugs, make sure your partner commits to administering Naloxone if you overdose.

However, Naloxone only works if you have a buddy with whom you are doing drugs. If you are getting high alone or locked in your room, you cannot administer Naloxone to yourself if you pass out and start to overdose. The best way to stay safe—other than not using drugs—is to test the drugs before taking them. We refer to these as fentanyl test strips. Don't rush out and buy these strips online, as you don't know their accuracy. It is best to seek advice from gay men's health organizations to determine which test strips are the best to buy. How do these test strips work? Put a small amount of the drug you're going to take in water, mix it, and dip the strip. The strip will display the potency of the fentanyl and any contaminants that could cause an overdose. Avoid taking any fentanyl-containing drugs, as they can lead to overdose. Bottom line: If you test any drug that reveals fentanyl, flush it down the toilet immediately. Yes, you are wasting money, but trust me, it's worth it. You don't want to risk an overdose, and you especially don't want to become addicted to fentanyl.

There are a variety of reasons why drug use is so rampant. The leading cause is peer pressure and the need to feel accepted by the gay community. Especially with Twinks (younger gay men), drug usage is a popular trend within the social context of being young, out, and gay. When you consume these drugs, you experience a profound high that leaves you feeling like you could dance all night long. However, some men use drugs for entirely different reasons. They do not feel like they fit into the gay community. So, they use drugs to numb their pain instead of facing their demons.

On the one hand, they carry this enormous sense of isolation. However, they also experience intense lust for another man. These men can temporarily feel wonderful about becoming intimate with another man by getting high—without anxiety, self-questioning, or guilt. It is just a temporary escape from the pain and misery. For the remaining drug users, getting high serves as a means to connect with their fellow users. As a result, it exposes these men to a large number of homeless addicts.

The drug use at the baths happens very late at night, courtesy of Twinks, who party hard and into the night. They begin the night by taking a hit of some drug. It seems to be a general rule that starting the evening without a buzz is impossible. Then they go from the clubs to the bars. They gather with their companions and persist in consuming more alcohol and drugs as they dance through the night. The bars close early in the morning, and many gay men head to the baths. But they aren't there to sleep it off. It is a post-party, a somewhat risky, sexually explicit post-party.

After midnight, many bathhouses turn the music on at full blast (to discourage sleepovers). However, for many who are high, hearing that loud, gyrating dance music has the opposite effect. The music seems to get everyone in the mood to continue the party. These men are so high on different combinations of drugs and alcohol that high-risk sex is not unusual. Crystal Meth (mixed with fentanyl) and Crack Cocaine will cause the user to experience such intense sexual euphoria that it becomes impossible to imagine engaging in sexual activity without feeling high. Being so high frees gay men from the burdensome worry of practicing safe sex. At that point, they can recreate the freewheeling days of the 1960s and 1970s. They can have sex with anyone and do anything without worrying about the consequences.

Despite the abundance of free-spirited sexual activity, it is not uncommon to observe men in public taking another dose of Crystal Meth or GHB (which is highly addictive). They are feeling high and do not care what people think. You often witness guys bouncing off the walls, high on substances, or passing out on one of the lounge chairs during the early morning hours. At the same time, you may hear scores of men engaging in group sex in their rooms. The bathhouse staff really cannot monitor what is going on. As the line outside the bathhouse continues to grow longer, the staff becomes excessively occupied with checking people out and turning over rooms. After 2 AM is the most active and best moneymaking time for the baths. The bars and clubs close, so the party must continue somewhere. You may ask why a bathhouse will let these intoxicated men enter. The desk attendant typically refuses entry to anyone who appears to be under the influence. So, to get around that rule, these Twinks take a different approach. They purchase a room before going out to club-hop. This ensures they won't face refusal upon their return, as they've already made their payment. Plus, they need not worry about getting a room if the bathhouse becomes 100% booked later in the evening. They secured their spot by paying in advance.

The 2 AM crowd also consists of men who have failed to find a partner at the bars. These guys have been hanging out at these taverns all night, looking for someone to pick up. If they fail to take someone home by closing time, they go to the gay baths to have sex with anyone they can find. Around 3 or 4 AM, the crowd transforms into a mix of club-hopping Twinks and middle-aged bar-type men eager to engage in sexual activities. No wonder a lineup always stretches around the corner at 2 a.m. every morning.

These younger gay men, exhausted from partying and non-stop sex, finally retire to their purchased room to sleep. But unfortunately, they wake up in a stupor sometime in the afternoon. Some even wake up finding someone unfamiliar in their bed. It is even worse if four or five guys are in your bed, and you have no idea how they got there. Though these Twinks are tired, sore, and strung out, they are ready to do it again. But most of these hardcore party guys know their limits. They have jobs, pay rent, and are aware of their responsibilities. By Monday morning, they are exhausted and need the rest of the week to recuperate. So why does it take a week to recover from a weekend of partying?

Long-term use of Crystal Meth can damage serotonin neurons in the brain. Serotonin is a critical neurochemical that regulates mood, emotion, learning, memory, sleep, and pain. Crystal meth can injure serotonin neurons, causing a variety of behavioral and cognitive consequences and impairing memory. After a weekend of partying, the drugs have fried the serotonin in your brain, leaving you in a daze. Although serotonin can regenerate, it is not a natural process and may not grow back. Many young gay men limit their partying to weekends. But for some, it has gotten out of hand, which is the dark side of gay bathhouses. This is the second part of the essay.

CHAPTER 10
Drug Use At The Gay Baths Part 2

The prevalence of drug use among gay men continues to amaze me. Many of these men can function, hold a job, and maintain relationships with others. Simultaneously, the individual is ingesting drugs all day long. They do not use marijuana or poppers. They consume hardcore drugs like GHB, Special K, speed, and even magic mushrooms. Drug use now seems to be the norm in mainstream gay culture. Certain gay elitist circles accept it and even consider it fashionable. While some men can handle these drugs, an equal number of gay men cannot. Inevitably, these men find their lives spinning out of control.

Let's focus on the darker side of the baths. You can quickly transition from being a recreational user to an addict. As an addict, your sole purpose is to scrape enough money to get high. If you're not a millionaire, this presents numerous challenges. Addicts lose themselves in a haze of alcohol, pot, crack, crystal meth, and anything else they can find. They become human garbage pails. I've even heard of someone so addicted to Crystal Meth that he wiped out all his savings and his kid's college fund, sold his condo, and stole money from other people to continue his habit. Now he's in hiding because he owes money (lots of it) to his drug dealer. Using this person's story as an example, it should be no surprise that many addicts become homeless. Where do they wind up? The Gay Baths, of course.

How do these addicts wind up living on and off at the baths? Most of these men had a successful life before they became addicted to drugs. They had jobs, friends, a home, and family. Regrettably, the experimentation with illegal substances ruined their lives. It starts with recreational drug use. Then it spirals out of control, leading to the onset of addiction. These men become drug addicts, consumed with the obsession of getting high. They have sold all their possessions for drugs and are now homeless. These addicts crash at the baths, but only when they have the money. Some of these addicts who stay at the baths are even straight. Beggars cannot be choosers when it comes to a roof over one's head.

Then there are the guys that are new to the scene. Everyday scores of young, twenty-something gay men arrive in the big city, all with a similar story. They have come from small towns or other states that do not have much of a gay community. Newly graduated from university, they cannot wait to arrive in the big metropolis and begin their new life. Others are teenagers who have run away from oppressive home lives, wanting to be free and gay.

Parents may also throw teenagers out of the house because of their queer identity. They've all had to flee their abusive home environments.

Whatever their story is, all these men arrive in the city with some optimism. Finally, they will be able to be amongst other gay men and feel part of a community. They are breaking out of their shells and embracing their freedom. Sounds romantic? However, it's important to exercise caution when making wishes, as they may come true. It is always the same with these young men. They arrive with a few thousand dollars in their pockets and big dreams in their heads. They have this romantic feeling that everything will be beautiful. However, after six months, you notice a dramatic change in these once optimistic men—a change that is not flattering. When they first arrive, they are fresh-faced with firm bodies, a bit naive with wide-eyed innocence. However, six months later, they look strung out, and their eyes appear fully dilated, as though they have visited an eye specialist.

If you are new to the "gay ghetto" and don't know anyone, you risk falling into the wrong crowd. The rent in the "gay ghetto" is enormous, with the first and last month's payment required to secure any place. These newbies find the cheapest place to spend the night—the bathhouse. They are filled with trepidation and fear because of the unfamiliarity of the place. They must choose between going to the baths or sleeping on the streets. The newbies will inevitably run into hustlers and drug users when they stay at the baths. With no friends, these newcomers want to fit in and make friends. Unfortunately, they will succumb to the drug scene and ultimately become addicts. Sometimes it occurs by happenstance; a newbie will meet a drug user, talk, and share a hit. Or, more likely, a drug dealer will target a newbie and deliberately get him high. Once the high becomes the person's only craving, there's no turning back. They become addicts.

While the bathhouse I regularly frequent is drug-free, not all baths are like that. Some bathhouses have drug dealers roaming the hallways looking to sell. As I wrote about gay prostitution earlier, a bathhouse can do nothing to stop this drug trafficking. Bathhouses are all about the privacy between two consenting adults. There is no way for a bathhouse to monitor what goes on in a private room. A drug dealer, as an added precaution, finds it wise to provide a free sample to a staff member in exchange for his silence. The dealer then goes to work, walking up and down the halls in search of men who want to get high or stay high. These dealers try to be discreet and conduct their business behind closed doors. But to maintain any business, drug dealers continually target the fresh, young newbies on the scene. The dealer will strike up a conversation with this newcomer. He will give the newbie a tiny bump as a welcome gift, just enough to get him hooked. The sooner the dealer can get a new addict hooked, the more money he makes. Inevitably, the dealer will have a new customer to add to his long list of clients.

Many of these drug users become homeless. But somehow, they scrape up enough money for a 12-hour room at the baths, so at least they have a place to sleep at night. Plus, the 12-hour room gives them "exit and re-entry" privileges to go out, score some drugs, and then return to the baths and get high in the privacy of their rented room. Inevitably, the gay baths become home to many of these homeless addicts. They all carry a knapsack containing their drug paraphernalia, a change of clothes, and some toiletry items (which they regularly shoplift, preferring to spend their money on drugs). The gay baths have all of the comforts of a home. There are showers, free liquid soap to stay clean, a television, a bed to sleep in, and a snack bar to buy food. Some baths even have a complimentary buffet once a week, and many homeless addicts make sure they are present for that. At some bathhouses, they even get their clothes washed and dried. The floor attendant throws their items in the washing machine, along with the towels and bedding that also need cleaning. However, not all floor attendants will be that nice. Some demand money or a sample of drugs in exchange, so a bribe is not uncommon.

What I have described may sound quaint, but trust me, it is not. As a drug addict, you find yourself involved in a community of other addicts. They all engage in deceit, theft, and strategizing to achieve that high. Observing all these hustlers, drug addicts, and drug dealers under the same roof is fascinating. At times it's almost like watching a soap opera, seeing them all interact with one another. These folks may appear, on the surface, to be friendly with one another. But they are far from being real friends. In reality, they could not care less about each other. They lack any feelings of jealousy, competitiveness, or threat. They all want to get high, which is the only thing on their minds.

Being addicted to drugs makes you lose track of time. The days and weeks have no structure, as the only thing that consumes an addict's mind is the prospect of getting high. It is not unusual for a drug addict to spend weeks at the baths because their drug dealer is there, so why bother leaving? I have even heard of one addict who spent an entire month inside the baths without ever going out. He was getting high daily. If you spend all your waking hours trying to score a hit, you have no time for a job. So, you do what other drug users do to score some quick cash. You sell your body for money, also known as hustling.

Prostitution and baths appear to be closely related. So, why do bathhouses tolerate hustling? Some bathhouse owners view prostitution as beneficial for their bottom line. If a gay man enters, hires a hustler, has sex, and then leaves, that customer can leave within 30 minutes. The more men come in and out, the more money the baths can make. Consequently, drug users often hustle to make a profit at the baths, with at least half of them being straight! It's not surprising that some addicts, once high, never leave the baths. They can sell their bodies for money and buy drugs at the baths to stay high. Taking all these drugs seems to make an addict's body razor-thin, a trait that appeals to men seeking sexual relations. I've always wondered how some hustlers had skinny bodies yet never went to the gym. Ecstasy speeds up a person's metabolism, as it is an amphetamine. If they take GHB, that stimulates the release of growth hormones, which act like an anabolic steroid. Therefore, addicts can achieve a muscular physique without engaging in any physical activity. So, they are ready for business.

They move from room to room, seeking companionship while discreetly claiming to be "working." Typically, they can lure a lonely married

Asian man for a 20-dollar blowjob. They can also offer a 60-dollar anal encounter to an elderly white man. They also target extremely obese men. Addicts understand that these three "types" of men are the most desperate for sex. They aim to spend as little time as possible with their mark. The only thing they want is money to buy more drugs. Desperation for money often leads these addicts to bargain down their prices. In the beginning, he may ask 40 dollars for a blowjob. The price has now fallen to $20 and then to $15. These men are willing to go to extreme measures to secure money for their drug addiction. Even during sexual encounters, a drug addict's primary concern is the amount of money they can earn from their drugs. It's how male addicts who are 100% straight manage to get through performing a blowjob, continuously imagining the drugs they get afterwards.

If an addict is unable to earn any money after attempting all the strategies I just discussed, they may resort to theft as a means of securing their drugs. If a bathhouse customer becomes a robbery victim, will they call the police? No, as it is embarrassing. Plus, look where the theft occurred—at a gay bathhouse. The most common theft occurs when two addicts' team up to steal money from an unsuspecting customer. One addict will likely distract their target, while the other will steal the customer's key and raid their room. Neither addict trusts the other to bring back equal amounts of drugs, so they both score the hit together. Alternatively, the addict may use GHB to induce unconsciousness in their victim. The addict will slip GHB into a customer's drink and wait for him to pass out. Once that happens, the addict takes the customer's money for drugs. I even heard a story where the addict used GHB to lubricate his dick. The customer sucked the addict's penis, rendering him unconscious.

When selling their body or stealing proves unsuccessful, they resort to begging as a final option. I have often seen these men pleading with customers for money at the baths. These addicts justify their actions by citing their impending locker termination due to overtime. The drug user initially breaks down in tears. He will swear that after he pays for the room and everything is alright, he will go to the nearest ATM and pay back the money. It is only a 5-minute loan, the drug user says. But in reality, it is for drugs, and once the user gets his money, he will claim the ATM was out of order! The scammed customer will never see his money again. The addict smoked it all away.

While I have described a bleak picture, not all baths are like this. The bathhouse I go to has a zero-tolerance policy on drugs and prostitution. They keep a list of drug addicts, dealers, and hustlers banned from the premises. Some bathhouses even refuse to offer exit and re-entry privileges. That is to curtail men from leaving the baths to score drugs, then returning to light up in the privacy of their rooms. Other bathhouses do not offer matches to their patrons. If an addict doesn't have a lighter, he can't light up behind closed doors. But let's be honest. Though the bathhouse I visit tries to be drug-free, you can't stop it. Drug use happens in every single bathhouse worldwide.

These addicts live in a never-ending cycle. Unfortunately, many gay establishments struggle to prevent drug use from occurring within their premises. As long as it is socially acceptable amongst gay men, overdoses like those I wrote about will continue. For these men, nothing is sacred.

CHAPTER 11
Gay Sex In The Dark Room

Every time I go to the gay baths, I always hope to meet someone I can make a connection with. Even for a brief period, I aspire to establish a physical and mental bond with someone. But after years of going to the baths, I realize I am in the minority. Most guys strongly desire quickie sex. Although quickies are a way of life for most gay men, I personally cannot indulge in them. As I mentioned in a previous essay, many guys do not want to give themselves totally to another person in a bathhouse. Men want to save that sexual connection for someone they genuinely care about (a future boyfriend or date). So, a quickie is a wonderful way for many guys to satisfy themselves and get off. Now you may read this and think quickie sex is degrading. However, in a bathhouse setting, anything is acceptable, which can lead to a desensitization to quickie sex, especially when it's so dark you can't see anything. This brings us to the realm of sex in the shadows. Men often make decisions based on their sexual desires rather than their rational thinking.

Any bathhouse you go to will have some mood lighting. If you have all the lights on in a bathhouse, the feeling is rather clinical and cold. Bathhouses install lighting to create a magical atmosphere. Some places have hallways lit a certain way, so there are dark corners everywhere you turn. In comparison, other baths will use special neon lighting to create a red glow (like a Red-Light District). I have even been in some bathhouses with special lighting effects, making towels worn by customers fluorescent white. As a result, the towels stand out in their semi-darkness.

Every bathhouse tries to create an atmosphere that is a throwback to days gone by. In the past, baths were considered a taboo subject. You go from the brightness of the day to the darkness of a bathhouse. It is like stepping into another world. It is so dark that you start bumping into things. But eventually, your eyes adjust to the darkness.

Because of the darkness, customers usually cannot see what is before them. While I can appreciate the mood within the bathhouse walls, I still cannot understand why it has to be that dark, as it is difficult to see all the adorable guys walking around. This is particularly frustrating for those who visit the baths seeking visual stimulation (eye candy).

Any bathhouse contains pockets of completely dark areas. Your eyes adjust to see shadows and figures moving in the dark. However, by and large, you cannot see anything. It forces you to rely on your sense of feeling. This allows you to evaluate the current situation.

Most bathhouses have what is known as a darkroom. These rooms feature everything from Glory Holes to open booths like telephone booths. Men enter these rooms, sizing up potential partners for quickies. Rarely is there any kissing—only anal and oral. Sex occurs while standing up or bending over. Amidst all the moans and grunts, the smell of amyl nitrate fills the air. There could be anywhere from two people getting together (because they do not have a private room and want to have sex) to a group having an orgy (four or five people, usually waiting around the darkroom for something to happen). Being in the dark adds mystery to sex because you have no idea what the other person looks like.

This is where the darkroom contradicts itself. Guys are notorious for being picky with their hookups. There is a high standard for getting laid, and the baths are no different. Very rarely will someone come in and immediately hit pay dirt. Instead, men prefer to wait for the right guy. This often results in them spending a significant amount of time waiting, cruising, lying in their room, and observing other guys. Some men go to the darkroom only out of sheer boredom and horniness. Who's waiting for those guys to arrive? The gay community's "have-nots."

The darkroom is an area of the baths that consists of men who can't score; Asians, obese men, and gay senior citizens—all of them lurking in the darkroom, waiting for something to happen. The darkness makes them unrecognizable, so no one will reject them! The dark makes all men equal and desirable. On Friday and Saturday nights, particularly after the bars close, these rooms are most crowded with horny men. These men want action—any action. Walking into the darkroom, sometimes you need to wear ten-inch-high boots. With so much semen on the floor, you don't know what you're stepping on.

Then it happens. The 72-year-old man is now accepting a blowjob from men who would not give these have-nots the time of day under the regular lighting of the baths. Because it is dark, he doesn't know who is sucking. However, this situation is filled with irony. Group action does take place. The darkroom at the baths is the closest equivalent to group sex. When two guys get it on in the dark, a few other guys may hear the grunts and join in. Before you know it, group sex is taking place, despite not knowing the looks of the other participants. It could be a 65-year-old grandfather or a 23-year-old college student. It doesn't really matter, as your primary goal is to satisfy your sexual desire. But let's be clear. If all lights were on, this group action wouldn't happen. Since guys are picky about who they hook up with, group sex in dark rooms means all players are desperate for sexual activity.

Occasionally, I've ventured into the darkroom and felt another guy's body against mine. You don't know how often I've touched an enormous belly or wrinkled skin. Knowing this is not someone I would generally hook up with, I'm not too fond of the darkroom because I want to know and see the person. But everyone is different.

While every bathhouse has a darkroom, many other places also have what is known as the "Dungeon Room." If a guy wants to experiment with S&M but does not have the proper equipment, they can visit the baths. It allows gay men to act out their fantasies with items on hand, such as swings, whips, leather, bondage equipment, and prison cells in the dungeon room for experimentation. I have seen many couples come to the baths together to act out their fantasies and have a wonderful time. In a controlled environment, they can play safely. Now, not all bathhouses have S&M equipment, so you should call ahead.

With the orgy and dungeon rooms being enormously popular with many men, some gay bathhouses have seized on that appeal by hosting a Blackout Night. The entire bathhouse plunges into darkness, with all lights turned off. Again, your eyes adjust to the complete darkness, but you still find yourself bumping into walls, furniture, and even people (hopefully friendly ones). Perhaps we should rename Blackout Night as Orgy Night, as it encompasses a large group of guys engaging in activities with each other. Although some light comes from the emergency exit signs and TV screens, it is still pitch dark. Every customer gets a small flashlight so you can navigate through the hallways, but that is it. Some places do not even offer these devices. Instead, they give out neon necklaces to indicate your preference. The red necklace is for those who identify as Top. At the same time, the green necklace is for those who identify as bottom. As customers look at the chain's color and choose their liking, communication is unnecessary. Blackout nights are so popular that some clubs host one every month. It is their biggest moneymaker, as scores of gay men line up around the block. Some bathhouses have enjoyed so much popularity from these events that they have kept the light shut off permanently, becoming known as the dark bathhouse.

Now, you can also use the darkness to your advantage. In a bathhouse, all rooms have light switches that allow you to dim the lights. The customer controls how bright or dark they want their room to be. Some men will rent a room, lie on a bed with the door open, and observe men passing by. But the customer keeps the lights turned off. So, all anyone sees is a darkened room, not the person inside. There are several reasons for this phenomenon. One reason could be the guy's desire to screen potential hookups. Although the room is dark, he can see everyone passing by. Those he deems unworthy of his time likely want to avoid bothering him. Those passing by his room should try to squint in order to see who's inside. It is so dark that men passing by cannot see anything. Again, it is a way to be selective and screen potential hook-ups. I remember seeing a couple intertwined on a bed, watching the men pass by their room. They came to the baths together, searching for a "threesome." Whenever anyone "undesirable" (in their minds, I guess) approached or even passed by their room, one of the guys would shut off the lights, making it pitch dark. This couple, I believe, was sending a clear message: "NO."

But another reason some guys keep their rooms dark is to hide parts of their bodies that they are embarrassed about. With the shadows and darkness obscuring their bodies, they feel more confident. But their minds are open to doing business. Entering someone's pitch-black room blindly can present certain challenges. Some guys may decide to chance it and enter the room. They are unaware of the guy's physical appearance. However, much like in the orgy room, they engage in sexual activity with their dicks rather than their minds. Some who can't see the other person will stand by the door, playing with themselves to gauge interest. They also try to get a better look at the guy. If the dude in the darkened room is uninterested, he will say, "No thanks." But if there is interest, he can say, "Come on in." So while that is an excellent screening process, not everybody likes it. Some guys who pass by dark rooms will keep walking without breaking stride—why buy what they can't see? These men are selective, which is why you won't find them in these dark rooms. They are selective and want to see what they can get. So, if you keep your room dark, you could miss out on someone kind, friendly, intelligent, or maybe a millionaire passing by your doorway, and vice versa!

So, am I scared of the darkness in the baths? Only when I am alone!

CHAPTER 12
Eye Contact At The Gay Baths

As you stroll down the street, the eye of a man catches yours. You don't pause to continue the gaze with a nod and a friendly smile; instead, you keep walking. While grocery shopping, your eyes meet another guy's briefly before you look away. At the gym, there were so many guys with so many eyes. However, you either keep your head down or look directly past everyone, thereby avoiding eye contact. Whether intentional or not, eye contact is a natural occurrence for every gay man out there. However, eye contact often triggers a superficial thought that many gay men experience, leading them to believe they are being hit on. Why does the act of making eye contact, being friendly, and acknowledging the other guy cause him to feel as though he is being hit on?

They say the eyes are a window to a person's soul. It is a way for two people to become intimate at a distance. Maintaining eye contact with someone is, in and of itself, a language. Most gay men use eye contact as their primary language, whether consciously or subconsciously. Gay men are prone to this behavior, as it's deeply ingrained in our DNA. However, eye contact could lead to the irrational sensation of scrutiny by other gay men, be it on the street, in a bank, at a supermarket, in a gym, or elsewhere. These are everyday situations where eye contact can happen. It seems that many guys will avoid eye contact and adopt this "pissed off" look on their faces most of the time. That look conveys the message to other guys: "Do not come near me," "Do not approach me," and "I am not interested." But in reality, that look masks the vast insecurity that almost all gay men carry, low self-esteem.

Recently, I've started sitting right in front of the main bathhouse entrance. That way, I can see which new customers are arriving at the baths. 85% of the men that enter avoid all eye contact with me. There is no acknowledgment, nod, or even a 'Hi.' Since the baths are known for their anonymity, that's a given. However, there are some guys I've seen at the baths for years. Walking in, they turn their heads and avoid looking at me altogether. Despite the fact that I am sitting directly in front of them, they still avoid looking at me.

I'm not cruising, chasing, or even threatening anyone. I'm just sitting there. What is so threatening about that? However, these guys avoid eye contact, indicating that they struggle with self-esteem, a common trait among gay men. You might be thinking, 'Well, maybe he is shy?' No. Shy people would need more guts to enter a place like the baths. I'm recognizable because I sit in the same spot week after week. Self-confident men wouldn't even feel the slightest bit of threat from me. They would give me a nod, a hello, or even stop to chat. The guys who avoid eye contact or even the slightest acknowledgment of me have issues. That individual exhibits low self-esteem.

Let's talk about eye contact in cruising locations. Whether you like it or not, eye contact is the language you use to assess a guy. There's no better place than the baths to exercise your eye contact skills with someone you like. The eyes speak, so there is little direct communication. I've received many letters from men complaining that no one approaches them at the baths. But eye contact is the best way to see whether the other person is interested. If I encounter a man who is of interest to me but fails to make eye contact and appears to be looking straight ahead, I am aware that this individual has no interest in me. I do not have to waste my time chasing this person; I can move on to someone else. Additionally, I am aware that the individual is conveying a message to other men to avoid him when he appears to be angry.

I recall encountering a **GORGEOUS** and **MUSCULAR** blond man who resembled a porn star. He kept his jeans on, but he was shirtless and wore sunglasses. It was summer, and during that time, the baths felt more like a pool house. Men would enter and exit the outdoor patio. They would be completely naked or be wearing a towel, having spent their time swimming or tanning (yes, the bathhouse I go to does allow nude tanning and swimming!). The blond guy stood in the hallway for an hour without getting any action. Finally, he approached me, recognizing my approachable face, and asked me what was wrong with all these guys. Excuse me, I said. He told me he was from out of town, and he dropped in to check out the bathhouse situation in my city. He couldn't understand what was wrong with all of the local guys. Why wasn't anyone approaching him? I explained that because he was wearing sunglasses, no one could make eye contact to see where his interest lay. Wearing jeans, he conveys a non-approachable demeanor and is likely only seeking a blow job. Given his attractive appearance and impressive physique, many men mistakenly believe he is beyond their reach. "I am unapproachable" was the signal he was projecting. He thought briefly about what I said and then replied, "Nah, it must be the guys here." With that, he left to go to another bathhouse. However, his demeanor conveyed the message, "I should not engage in conversation until I approach you."

I recall a different, stunning individual in the porn room who sported a full erection at the baths. He stroked himself up and down, all ripe and ready to receive oral. It looks like he wanted anyone to give him a blow job, right? **WRONG!** Whenever anyone even entered the porn room, this gorgeous guy would shoot daggers with his eyes. His eyes conveyed a powerful message to all of us: "Leave immediately." I guess he was hoping for someone more to his liking, whatever those standards may be.

But I can't stand guys who go out of their way to avoid me. Even after I have gotten the message that they have no interest in me, I leave them alone. I must acknowledge my sensitivity and thin skin. However, I find it personally hurtful when someone avoids me. Examples include exiting a room when I enter, taking a different route in the hallways to steer clear of me, and even walking the long way around the halls so passing my room doesn't happen. It is challenging to desensitize yourself from that type of blatant rejection. I know I should not take it personally, but it is hard. What else are they rejecting—the chair I'm sitting in? Are they rejecting the towel I'm wearing? Of course not; they're rejecting me. But I can also understand them acting that way. Many Asian men have developed a habit of repeatedly making advances toward white men. I regularly witness this behavior at gay baths. After being approached by numerous Asian men, many gay men tend to label all gay Asians as desperate and pursue them relentlessly.

I hate it when guys act arrogantly and presume they are the center of attention, thinking, "All these stares are exhausting." In reality, they are average in appearance and often go unnoticed by others. It is especially true for overweight and out-of-shape men who run into Asians in the hallways. As I previously stated, the stereotype of Asians pursuing gay white men leads these guys to believe we are pursuing them! Thus, they turn their heads, look away, and emit an attitude when any Asian male enters a room, as if we would be interested in them. Forget about just having a conversation with someone cute. Men perceive eye contact in the lounge as a form of harassment, as previously mentioned. Therefore, they avoid conversations to stop the other person from 'cruising' them.

Conversely, I have encountered situations where older men in their sixties have pursued me to the extent of stalking. Although it pains me to do so, I must resort to the behavior I've discussed in order to distance myself from these older men. These older men seem to lack the ability to accept rejection. Sometimes, an older man stands outside my room, trying to make eye contact with me while massaging his cock. To demonstrate my disinterest, I look away, turn my head, and stare at the ceiling, all in the hopes of showing that I have no interest. Usually, that works. On several occasions, I've looked away for over five minutes, but the older guy hasn't given up. At this point, I will usually say, 'I am just resting.' The older guy leaves, but he continues to cruise and watch me for the remainder of my stay.

One time I was in the whirlpool, and this 70-year-old man got in and sat near me. I was not interested, and I tried to make that transparent. I sat away from him, positioned myself to face a wall, and curled up in a fetal position. You would think that he would understand the message. But what did he do? Under the water, he tried to play footsie with me. I did not expect him to touch me, and when he did, I was so surprised that I yelled and sprang up! Then he took offense to my outburst. Excuse me, but who was cruising whom? Is it not obvious from my actions that I am not interested? But of course, you all know my theory of why older guys chase after Asians.

It upsets me that I have to treat these older gentlemen this way because of my job at the Gay Elder Center. Unfortunately, there are times when it's necessary to be direct and express disinterest. However, many older men approach me for conversation because I am very approachable. I always tell the older men this is just conversation.

While I've seen regulars at the baths who don't talk to me, I always attempt to acknowledge the person with some eye contact and a nod. Some guys appreciate the acknowledgment and return with a nod. Others look right past me without even a second glance. I always say hello when I encounter someone I've hooked up with. But only some guys do that. Usually, they act as if they have never seen you before. Guys who do this are dealing with their own insecurities and problems. However, not all men behave in this manner. When I've crossed paths with some men, our nods transform into hellos and then into conversations.

For four years, I've seen one guy my age at the baths every Saturday afternoon. If there were Saturday afternoon regulars, it would be the two of us. It took years for us to nod and greet each other. Now, we engage in brief conversations about things like the weather. That is because we have seen each other so many times. Friendships at the baths are tenuous and superficial. I sometimes wonder about him, what makes him tick, and why he comes to the baths. We may go for coffee outside the bathhouse and learn more about each other. I will have to keep you posted.

CHAPTER 13
The Politics of Gay Oral Sex

Oral sex is the most common sex act at the baths; you can see it everywhere. There is a significant amount of oral sex taking place in the whirlpool, shower area, and lounge. It is so commonplace that it seems to be a prerequisite to be a gay man—that you must participate in oral sex.

When people think of oral sex, most envision this personal, intimate bonding experience between two people who genuinely care for each other. You have the opportunity to fully give yourself to another person. However, gay men need to break free from the heterosexual mindset. Oral sex is not sacred in the gay community. Kissing is the equivalent of displaying intimate contact between two men. You can get a blow job anywhere. Guys want to save real, physical, and close contact, such as kissing, for a future boyfriend. Many men have told me they do not even kiss guys they may encounter at the baths. Oral sex? No problem. Anal? Pass the lube. But kissing? NO WAY! You would expect the situation to be reversed.

For instance, I've seen this one Caucasian guy at the baths for the past few years. I've spoken to him several times; he is gay, amiable, and cute! However, the sole activity he enjoys at the baths is performing blowjobs, and he has no other interests. He avoids kissing, hugging, and anal contact. He focuses solely on delivering oral sex to one individual after another. I think his record is fifty blowjobs in one night. He doesn't discriminate between races, ages, or the person's weight. I've seen him go from Black to White, fat to thin, old to young—just a variety of men. He only cares about the cock's size. I guess that's one reason I've never seen him suck an Asian cock.

On a regular basis, I've seen this other young, white guy at the baths. My opinion is that he identifies as straight but suppresses his desire for men. Whenever these cravings become overwhelming, he drops by the baths. I've seen him multiple times, at all hours of the day. All he does is give blowjobs every chance he gets. Once, I watched him become so engrossed in the act of sucking cock that he would slurp it as if it were his last meal, refusing to stop. The man receiving the blowjob appeared to feel ensnared, with no alternative but to remain seated, persist in watching the pornographic film, and relish the sensation.

Gay men aren't the only ones who enjoy getting their cock sucked off. You can find many straight guys prowling the gay baths seeking a blowjob. They have wives, girlfriends, or even fiancées who don't like to perform oral sex on their significant other. Many women find it gross. So, what should a man do if he is not getting it at home? They go to the baths. Many straight men don't consider oral sex adultery or even sex. They see it as a way to get off. Here's a method for identifying a straight man in the gay baths who wants a blow job: The man would be fully clothed, the zipper undone, with his cock hanging out. It gives a new meaning to the phrase "Well Hung!"

I remember one guy whose sole purpose for going to the gay baths was to get oral sex. Every week, he consistently showed up at the baths on the same day and time. He would situate himself in the porn room and start stroking himself. Then a succession of over twenty guys would suck him for over three hours! During that time, he would never say anything. Some blowjobs lasted a minute; others could go on longer. After three hours, he would shower, get dressed, and leave. Men waited for him in the porn room because of his popularity and consistency. At least 70% of those guys were Asian!

There are also places known as "glory holes." Men insert their penis through an opening, then wait for a passerby to suck them off. On one side, the person receiving doesn't know who is doing the sucking. The person on the other side is unaware of whose cock it is. All the guy sees is a cock hanging out of a hole, so he goes for it. This is a place where sex is truly anonymous! There is even a "slurp ramp"! That's where men stand next to each other, all in a row, sticking their dicks through a hole. On the other side, men can suck off the cocks one after the other.

Therefore, if you're a guy who loves to give, there's no shortage of cocks to suck. However, based on what I have seen at the baths, guys are more inclined to receive than to give. You'll notice that every example I write about involves guys who prefer to receive rather than give. Oral sex, in my opinion, primarily revolves around a power dynamic (a cock staring you in the face). Instead of allowing things to unfold naturally, the other person dictates the course of action. Many gay Asians, often perceived as passive participants, are particularly susceptible to this phenomenon.

After decades of going to the baths, I still see gay Asian men giving heads to anyone and everyone in record numbers. It is a never-ending cycle. I seldom observe a gay Asian man at the baths decline to engage in oral sex with an individual, no matter the age, even 70. It's no surprise that many older gay men find Asians attractive! However, in reality, it is a self-esteem issue, as many gay Asian men lack self-confidence. As a result, gay Asians seek validation from gay white men, who are considered the standard in the gay community. Therefore, in order to validate themselves, one must engage with as many gay white men as possible. But I also genuinely believe many white guys at the baths view Asians as the ultimate "backup." During their stay at the baths, they hunt for good-looking prey. However, if they are unsuccessful in finding anyone, they turn their attention to the desperate Asian man who is waiting in the wings.

It disturbs me that gay men only see us Asians as a way to serve them, like some concubines freely giving out blowjobs. After receiving oral pleasure from an Asian, these gay white men depart. They do not express gratitude, acknowledgment, or even a nod. Once they are satisfied, these gay white men wrap their towel around their midsection and depart to seek out other men. Those Asians would be on their knees, still in position, with their mouths open, getting nothing. Unless the Asian in question genuinely enjoys giving blowjobs, the only satisfaction these Asian men experience is a fleeting sense of fulfillment when they blow a White man. But it is a vicious cycle for these Asians. After blowing a Caucasian man, many of them feel used. However, five minutes later, they are already looking for another white man to blow. They do this in order to continue receiving the validation they desire.

Despite the risks of HPV (oral cancer) and other STIs associated with oral sucking, no one is using a condom. Gay guys won't suck cock while wearing a condom. That will not happen. What if you're one of the rare guys who uses condoms for oral sex? It depends on the person and how things are progressing. You can say immediately, "I do not engage in oral sex without a condom." Most of the time, you will have guys who become incredulous and leave without saying a word.

Surprisingly, you might find the odd guy who will put the condom on. If he likes you, he'll do anything you ask. However, this is a rare occurrence. However, there are some instances where a man expresses no interest in oral sex, and other circumstances arise. Alternatively, he engages in giving oral sex without seeking reciprocation. Of course, there are instances where things escalate quickly without any established ground rules. Suddenly, you find yourself staring at an erect penis right in your face. That is when you would say, "I just brushed my teeth" or "I just came from the dentist." If the guy leaves, he leaves. If you take anything away from this essay, make sure it's this one. Vaccinate against HPV to lower your risk of developing oral cancer. Speak with your family doctor about the vaccination process.

While I have just written about the politics and etiquette around oral sex, there is one topic I have not covered. I have not addressed the topic of ejaculating into a man's mouth. It would be best to always ask **BEFOREHAND**. It is unacceptable to squirt into a guy's mouth without asking. Most guys consistently inquire whether they can ejaculate in the mouth or not. At the very least, they would give a warning, indicating that they were close. Cumming in someone's mouth without asking or warning is just unacceptable manners.

So, after writing about the politics of oral sex, I hope I've clarified things for anyone new to the ins and outs of blowjobs. Just because every gay man performs oral sex doesn't mean you should. It isn't for everyone. Don't feel pressured to do it for one minute. Remember what I always say: Don't do anything you are uncomfortable doing. Only you and no one else can know what's best for you.

CHAPTER 14
Making The Connection

For men who go to the baths, it is not just about sex. It's about making a connection—the desire for gay men to connect with other gay men.

Why is there this need to make a connection with someone? One word: loneliness, or rather, a subconscious feeling of isolation. Despite the strides and advances made by gays and lesbians in mainstream society, it still feels isolating to be "gay" in the gay community. Many men feel they don't fit in.

Having a lower status in the gay community exacerbates the situation. Gay men regularly criticize their peers, whom they perceive to be "lower class." Whether the person is of a different ethnicity or drives a used car, there is nothing anyone can do to change the elitist gay atmosphere. Remember, it's more about the individual expressing it than it is about demonizing the group. The problem lies with the snobby gay men. Many of those men have self-esteem and insecurity issues. So, they take it out on others in order to feel better about themselves. With the bars and clubs filled with pretentious and superficial gay men, where can gay men go to feel accepted? If you thought of the baths, you would be right.

The baths can be just as superficial as the bars and clubs. But it is also a place where everyone is on somewhat equal footing. Because everyone is naked in a towel, there is no class distinction. Lawyers interact with truck drivers, and so on. Plus, the baths are the only gay environment where you can see every type of gay man, regardless of age or race. Bathhouses are an environment where anonymity reigns supreme behind closed doors. While the connection you are making with someone else is a sexual one, underneath those sexual feelings lies the need to connect. Look at all of the numerous blowjobs that take place in sex clubs, bars, clubs, dance halls, and even public bathrooms. All this oral activity is, in reality, the need to connect with someone else, no matter how short or fleeting the experience may be.

For instance, I've seen this one Caucasian guy at the baths for the past few years. I've spoken to him several times; he is gay, amiable, and cute! However, the sole activity he enjoys at the baths is performing blowjobs, and he has no other interests. He avoids kissing, hugging, and anal contact. He focuses solely on delivering blowjobs to one individual after another. I think his record is fifty blowjobs in one night. He doesn't discriminate between races, ages, or the person's weight. I've observed him interacting with a diverse range of men—from Black to white, from fat to thin, from old to young—regardless of their race, age, or weight. I doubt he pays much attention to a man's physical appearance. He only cares about the cock and its size. I suppose that is one of the reasons I have never witnessed him perform oral on an Asian guy.

Then there is this other white guy, who I suspect identifies as straight but suppresses his desire for men. Whenever these cravings become overwhelming, he drops by the baths. I've seen him multiple times, at all hours of the day. All he does is give blowjobs every chance he gets. I once saw him performing oral sex on another guy for an hour! He was so engaged in sucking that cock that he slurped that dick like it was his last meal, refusing to stop. The man receiving the blowjob appeared to feel ensnared, with no alternative but to remain seated, persist in watching the pornographic film, and relish the sensation.

This straight guy is synonymous with the fact that you see more married, bi, or closeted men at the baths than in any other gay environment (like bars or clubs). These men rarely interact with the gay community, and their strong desire to connect with other gay men is evident. This need stems from their insecurity and denial about their sexuality. These men can fill that void of insecurity by interacting with other gays. Thus, they feel secure. However, this feeling of security is fleeting, as the need soon returns. The baths offer these men a false sense of security and acceptance. The baths provide these men with the liberty to release inhibitions and experience freedom beyond their daily routines. Since the baths are anonymous and closed-door, they feel safer connecting with other gay men. Baths offer anonymity, unlike bars and clubs, which are visible.

While these men have an overwhelming need to connect with other guys, they don't want to get too close. But that is the beauty of the baths. They can bond sexually with another man, and that encounter will remain anonymous and detached. There is only pure, raw sex; there is no conversation, no names exchanged, and no getting to know you. Once these men ejaculate, those pent-up feelings of loneliness evaporate. One quick shower, and he's on his merry way. But trust me, those feelings of loneliness resurface a few hours later. These men can't get back to the baths fast enough. For openly gay men, it just means more fun at the baths. However, for those who are closeted, it can be a frustrating cycle.

But it is not only straight men who need to connect; gay men have the same need. That is why many of the same men hang out at the baths all the time. It is almost like being a familiar face at the same bar night after night. Why are there so many gay bathhouse regulars? This is due to a subliminal sense of isolation and a yearning to establish connections with fellow gay men, similar to those in close relationships. The aim is to experience a feeling of inclusion in the gay community.

For instance, I have seen this good-looking Russian man at the baths every week. But how do I know he is Russian? He has shared his life story with anyone who will listen, complete with a heavy Russian accent. The Russian will approach any white guy and start a conversation about anything and everything. Occasionally, this Russian man might make a sexual connection as well. However, a warning: some guys find it annoying when strangers come up and start talking. For some men looking for pure sex, conversation just gets in the way.

I've overheard bits of his conversations with other white guys. I suspect he is still in the closet, as he also considers himself straighter than gay. Observing this Russian being sociable and engaging in conversation with every White man struck me as a desperate attempt to connect with the gay community. I've even heard the Russian admit to other men that he uses the baths to socialize. It allows him to meet other gay men, as he doesn't know where to meet them.

But another thing struck me about the Russian man. After a while, I couldn't help noticing that he never spoke to any people of color at the baths. He spoke to every Caucasian person, old or young, fat or thin. At the baths, he never spoke to me or other visible minorities. However, as soon as a Caucasian man appeared, the Russian would immediately engage in conversation. You could almost see the desperation in his eyes. Even in his body language, he wanted to connect with anyone—as long as they were white.

I know I'm speaking about the racial thing again. But it is only human nature to feel safe and secure around people like themselves. Therefore, a Caucasian Russian would likely find comfort only in the company of similar white individuals. Being in Russia doesn't expose him to many visible minorities. So, he probably feels a sense of 'foreignness' around anyone who isn't White. However, he also appeared to exhibit a strong sense of status consciousness, a trait I previously identified as common among gay men. This explains why he limits his communication and engagement to white men.

Asians are another class-conscious group. Yes, I'm on that subject again, but the following anecdote is too useful not to tell. The other day, I was at the baths and observed a twenty-something Asian man who was extremely muscular (and yes, the Russian man also ignored him!). He appeared quite agitated, walking up and down the halls impatiently. Eventually, they called his room number for either check-out or room renewal. But he wasn't ready to go. So, he checked out of his room and purchased a locker to stay longer. I later heard from the front desk attendant that he had been at the baths for 8 hours. He must have been desperate for some attention! As time went on, he became more and more bitchy. At least, that is what the bathhouse staff observed.

The next thing I knew, he checked out his locker, purchased another room, and was with a white hustler. All of a sudden, his personality changed. No longer was he rude and scowling at other people. As he bonded with his hired white hustler, he was filled with laughter and joy. However, the shocking truth is that they rarely engaged in sexual activity. They spent most of their time talking. I'm sure they had sex at some point. But it was almost like the Asian guy wanted and needed company and conversation, and it had to be from someone Caucasian.

This Asian guy has an inherent repressed inferiority complex, as if a conversation with a white guy is better than one with an Asian guy. I perceived him engaging in conversation with a white person as a means of social advancement. He aspired to 'improve' himself, akin to a gold digger. Look at the amount of money he spent in just one day. For all his time at the baths (over 12 hours) and renting that white guy just for conversation, it cost him about $400.00.

When I observe the Russian or the Asian guy, I see someone's overwhelming need to connect. They seek acceptance and a sense of belonging within the gay community. But what else is there to do besides go to the gay baths? The solution is to make that connection within yourself. Only through therapy can you achieve that feeling of contentment. Do that, and I guarantee it will be a wonderful feeling.

CONTACT BATHHOUSE BLUES

http://www.bathhouseblues.com